Endoscopic Ear Surgery

Editors

MUAAZ TARABICHI
JOÃO FLÁVIO NOGUEIRA
DANIELE MARCHIONI
LIVIO PRESUTTI
DAVID D. POTHIER

OTOLARYNGOLOGIC CLINICS OF NORTH AMERICA

www.oto.theclinics.com

April 2013 • Volume 46 • Number 2

ELSEVIER

1600 John F. Kennedy Boulevard • Suite 1800 • Philadelphia, Pennsylvania, 19103-2899

http://www.theclinics.com

OTOLARYNGOLOGIC CLINICS OF NORTH AMERICA Volume 46, Number 2
April 2013 ISSN 0030-6665, ISBN-13: 978-1-4557-7132-5

Editor: Joanne Husovski
Development Editor: Donald Mumford

Otolaryngologic Clinics of North America (ISSN 0030-6665) is published bimonthly by Elsevier, Inc., 360 Park Avenue South, New York, NY 10010-1710. Months of issue are February, April, June, August, October, and December. Business and Editorial Offices: 1600 John F. Kennedy Blvd., Suite 1800, Philadelphia, PA 19103-2899. Customer Service Office: 6277 Sea Harbor Drive, Orlando, FL 32887-4800. Periodicals postage paid at New York, NY and additional mailing offices. Subscription prices is $335.00 per year (US individuals), $628.00 per year (US institutions), $161.00 per year (US student/resident), $442.00 per year (Canadian individuals), $789.00 per year (Canadian institutions), $496.00 per year (international individuals), $789.00 per year (international institutions), $248.00 per year (international & Canadian student/resident). Foreign air speed delivery is included in all *Clinics*' subscription prices. All prices are subject to change without notice. **POSTMASTER:** Send address changes to *Otolaryngologic Clinics of North America*, Elsevier Health Sciences Division, Subscription Customer Service, 3251 Riverport Lane, Maryland Heights, MO 63043. **Telephone: 1-800-654-2452 (U.S. and Canada); 314-447-8871 (outside U.S. and Canada). Fax: 314-447-8029. E-mail: journalscustomerservice-usa@elsevier.com (for print support); journalsonlinesupport-usa@elsevier.com (for online support).**

Reprints. For copies of 100 or more of articles in this publication, please contact the Commercial Reprints Department, Elsevier Inc., 360 Park Avenue South, New York, NY 10010-1710. Tel.: 212-633-3812; Fax: 212-462-1935; E-mail: reprints@elsevier.com.

Otolaryngologic Clinics of North America is also published in Spanish by McGraw-Hill Interamericana Editores S.A., P.O. Box 5-237, 06500 Mexico D.F., Mexico.

Otolaryngologic Clinics of North America is covered in *MEDLINE/PubMed (Index Medicus), Current Contents/Clinical Medicine, Excerpta Medica, BIOSIS, Science Citation Index,* and *ISI/BIOMED.*

Printed and bound by CPI Group (UK) Ltd, Croydon, CR0 4YY

Transferred to digital print 2013

Contributors

AUTHORS

MATTEO ALICANDRI-CIUFELLI, MD
Department of Otolaryngology, Head and Neck Surgery, University Hospital of Modena, Modena, Italy

MUNAHI AL QAHTANI, MD
Department of Otolaryngology, Riyadh Military Hospital, Riyadh, Saudi Arabia

STÉPHANE AYACHE, MD
Chairman of ENT ENDOSCOPY Meeting, Department of Otolaryngology, Head and Neck Surgery, ORPAC; Private Hospital Center, Grasse; IWGEES (International Working Group on Endoscopic Ear Surgery), France

MOHAMED BADR-EL-DINE, MD
Professor of Otolaryngology, Department of Otolaryngology; President of the Egyptian Society of Skull Base Surgery; Consultant Otology, Neurotology and Skull Base Surgery, Faculty of Medicine, University of Alexandria, Alexandria, Egypt

ADRIAN L. JAMES, MA, DM, FRCS(ORL-HNS)
Associate Professor, Department of Otolaryngology—Head and Neck Surgery, Hospital for Sick Children, University of Toronto, Toronto, Ontario, Canada

SEIJI KAKEHATA, MD, PhD
Professor and Chairman, Department of Otolaryngology Head and Neck Surgery, Yamagata University Faculty of Medicine, Japan

DANIELE MARCHIONI, MD
Professor of Otolaryngology, Department of Otolaryngology, Facoltà di Medicina e Chirurgia, Università degli Studi di Modena e Reggio Emilia; Department of Otolaryngology, Head and Neck Surgery, University Hospital of Modena, Modena, Italy

FRANCESCO MATTIOLI, MD
Department of Otolaryngology, University Hospital of Modena, Modena, Italy

JOÃO FLÁVIO NOGUEIRA, MD
ENT Professor, Director of Sinus & Oto Centro, Department of Otolaryngology, Hospital Geral de Fortaleza, Fortaleza, Brazil; Instituto de Otorrinolaringologia e Oftalmologia de Fortaleza - IOF Sinus Centro, Fortaleza, Ceara, Brazil

GIUSEPPE PANETTI, MD
Consultant, Department of Otolaryngology, ASCALESI Hospital; National Counsellor of AOOI (Italian Association of Hospital Otolaryngologists), Chair of Audiology, Faculty of Medicine "Federico II" Naples, Naples, Italy

ALESSIA PICCININI, MD
Department of Otolaryngology, Head and Neck Surgery, University Hospital of Modena, Modena, Italy

DAVID D. POTHIER, MBChB, MSc, FRCS(ORL-HNS)
Neurotology Affiliate, Department of Otolaryngology, Head and Neck Surgery, Toronto General Hospital, University Health Network, University of Toronto, Toronto, Ontario, Canada

LIVIO PRESUTTI, MD
Professor, Department of Otolaryngology, University Hospital of Modena; Professor of Otolaryngology, Chairman, Department of Otolaryngology, Head and Neck Surgery, Facoltà di Medicina e Chirurgia, Università degli Studi di Modena e Reggio Emilia, Modena, Italy

MUAAZ TARABICHI, MD
Center for Ear Endoscopy, Kenosha, Wisconsin

DOMENICO VILLARI, MD
Department of Otolaryngology, University Hospital of Modena, Modena, Italy

Contents

ear inflammatory disorders during middle ear surgery; intraoperative evaluation of middle ear anatomy during endoscopic surgery for inflammatory disorders helps surgeon visualize anatomic blockages of the middle ear ventilation trajectories. This article discusses the anatomy of the epitympanum and the ventilation patterns and pathophysiology of epitympanic retraction.

OTOLARYNGOLOGIC CLINICS
OF NORTH AMERICA

NOW AVAILABLE FOR YOUR iPhone and iPad

Transcanal Endoscopic Management of Cholesteatoma

Muaaz Tarabichi, MD[a],*, João Flávio Nogueira, MD[b],
Daniele Marchioni, MD[c], Livio Presutti, MD[c],
David D. Pothier, MBChB, MSc, FRCS(ORL-HNS)[d], Stéphane Ayache, MD[e]

KEYWORDS

- Cholesteatoma • Endoscopy • Ear endoscopy • Surgical management
- Surgical approaches • Anatomy

KEY POINTS

- The endoscope offers a new perspective of cholesteatoma and related surgical procedures by increasing the surgeon's understanding of that disorder and its progression through the temporal bone.
- Rediscovering the ear canal as the access port for cholesteatoma surgery is the main story and the main advantage of endoscopic ear surgery. This approach allows a more natural and direct access to and pursuit of cholesteatoma within the middle ear cleft.
- Endoscopic Technique allows better access to the tympanic cavity, the birthplace of cholesteatoma, and allows the surgeon to identify the cause for any selective atelectasis or poor ventilation.
- The Endoscope allows better access for the tympanic cavity for removal of cholesteatoma especially within the retrotympanum, the anterior attic, anterior mesotympanum, and eustachian tube.
- The endoscope is of limited use within the mastoid cavity proper and disease within the mastoid is best eradicated using traditional microscopic approaches.

 Videos on transcanal endoscopic removal of cholesteatoma, endoscopic "Open Cavity" approach to cholesteatoma, endoscopic lateral canal approach to cholesteatoma and the isthmus ventilating the attic accompany this article at http://www.oto.theclinics.com/

A version of this article appeared in Tarabichi M, Marchioni D, Presutti L, et al. Transcanal Endoscopic Management of Cholesteatoma. Tuttlingen, Germany: Endo Press, 2011. Used with permission of Karl Storz GmbH & Co.
[a] Center for Ear Endoscopy, Kenosha, Wisconsin; [b] UECE – State University of Ceara, Fortaleza, Brazil; [c] Department of Otolaryngolgy, University Hospital of Modena, Modena, Italy; [d] Department of Otolaryngology-Head and Neck Surgery, University of Toronto, Toronto, Ontario, Canada; [e] Department of Otolaryngology, ORPAC, Clinique du Palais, Grasse, France
* Corresponding author.
E-mail address: tarabichi@yahoo.com

Otolaryngol Clin N Am 46 (2013) 107–130
http://dx.doi.org/10.1016/j.otc.2012.10.001
0030-6665/13/$ – see front matter © 2013 Elsevier Inc. All rights reserved.

INTRODUCTION

Although it has been 2 decades since the first use of operative endoscopy for the exploration of old mastoid cavities, the endoscope is used infrequently in the day-to-day surgical management of ear disease around the globe for several reasons.[1] The role of the endoscope as defined by many prominent otologists is so marginal that most surgeons have not felt compelled to master newer techniques and instrumentation for its use.[2–6] In effect, the use of the endoscope did not significantly benefit either the patient or the surgeon. In addition, most physicians have focused on the use of smaller diameter endoscopes for ear surgery, which is frustrating and eliminates the main (and possibly the only) advantage of endoscopy (the wide field of view provided by the endoscope is greater than that of the microscope). Our first experience of using the endoscope in ear surgery was in 1993 during years of practice in the United States. In recent years, it has replaced the microscope as the instrument of choice for use in middle ear surgery.[7–10] The endoscope offers a new perspective of cholesteatoma and related surgical procedures by increasing the surgeon's understanding of that disorder and its progression through the temporal bone. Clinicians who use the endoscope during ear surgery realize how the microscope and its limitations have colored the clinical perception of cholesteatoma and have dictated its management (Videos 1–3).

HISTORY

The introduction of the binocular operating microscope, which was a landmark event in the development of modern otology, clearly changed the scope and character of ear surgery. Despite continuous technical improvements, however, basic optical principles and their limitations have remained the same over the last the decades. The use of the endoscope in various surgical procedures was extrapolated to otologic surgery, and the diagnostic and photographic use of that instrument in the examination of the tympanic membrane and the ear canal has been widely publicized.[2] Transtympanic middle ear endoscopy was initially reported by Nomura[3] and Takahashi and colleagues.[4] Poe and Bottrill[5] used transtympanic endoscopy for the confirmation of perilymphatic fistula and the identification of other middle ear pathologic conditions. Kakehata and colleagues[11–13] used microendoscopy and transtympanic endoscopy for evaluation of conductive hearing loss and inspection of retraction pockets. Thomassin and colleagues[1] reported on operative ear endoscopy for mastoid cavities and designed an instrument set to be used for that purpose. Badr-el-Dine[14] and El-Messelaty and colleagues[15] reported on the value of endoscopy as an adjunct in cholesteatoma surgery and documented a reduced risk of recurrence when the endoscope was used. The reduction in residual disease was further confirmed by Yung[16] and Ayache and colleagues.[17] Abdel Baki and colleagues[18] reported on using the endoscopic technique to evaluate disease within the sinus tympani. Mattox[19] reported on endoscopy-assisted surgery of the petrous apex. Magnan and Sanna,[20] Bader-el-Dine and colleagues, El-Garem and colleagues,[21–23] and Rosenberg and colleagues[24] reviewed the role of the endoscope in neuro-otologic procedures. McKennan[6] described second-look endoscopic inspection of mastoid cavities achieved through a small postauricular incision. More recently, Presutti and colleagues[25] and Marchioni and colleagues[26] described primary transcanal endoscopic ear surgery using a similar approach to the experience reported here.

INSTRUMENTATION

In the procedures described in this article, 4-mm wide-angle 0-degree and 30-degree Hopkins II telescopes that were 18 cm in length were most often used. More recently, a smaller 3-mm endoscope with a similar field of view to the 4-mm endoscope is being used. Other smaller diameter scopes were used sparingly. Video equipment consisted of a 3-chip video camera and a monitor. All procedures were performed directly off the monitor and were recorded. Instruments used in conjunction with routine microscopic ear surgery are shown in **Fig. 1**.

DISCUSSION

The rationale advantages and limitations, and the technique and long-term results of endoscopic transcanal management of limited cholesteatoma, endoscopic open cavity management of cholesteatoma, and expanded transcanal access to the middle ear and petrous apex are discussed in the following sections.

Rationale for Endoscopic Ear Surgery

Acquired cholesteatoma is usually a manifestation of advanced retraction of the tympanic membrane, which occurs when the sac advances into the tympanic cavity proper and then into its extensions, such as the sinus tympani, the facial recess, the hypotympanum, and the attic.[27] Only in advanced cases does a cholesteatoma progress further to reach the mastoid cavity proper. Most surgical failures associated with a postauricular approach seem to occur within the tympanic cavity and its hard-to-reach extensions rather than in the mastoid.[28,29] Therefore, the most logical approach to the excision of a cholesteatoma involves transcanal access to the tympanic membrane and tympanic cavity and the subsequent step-by-step pursuit of the sac as it passes through the middle ear. Mainstream ear surgery has usually involved the mastoid and the postauricular approaches because operating with the microscope through the auditory canal is a frustrating and almost impossible process.

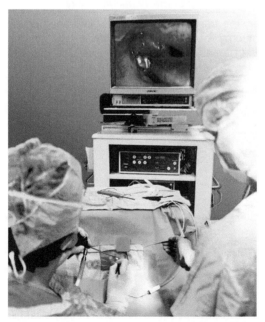

Fig. 1. Operating room setup. The surgeon is operating while watching the monitor, which is positioned across the operating room table. The surgical assistant also has a clear view of the monitor.

Advantages and Limitations

The view during microscopic surgery is defined and limited by the narrowest segment of the ear canal (**Fig. 2**). This basic limitation has forced surgeons to create a parallel port through the mastoid to gain keyhole access to the attic, the facial recess, and the hypotympanum (**Fig. 3**). In contrast, transcanal operative endoscopy bypasses the narrow segment of the ear canal and provides a wide view that enables surgeons to look around the corner, even when a 0-degree endoscope is used (see **Fig. 2**). Another anatomic observation that supports transcanal access to the attic, which is the most frequent site of cholesteatoma,[30] is the orientation of the ear canal in relation to the attic. **Fig. 4** shows a coronal computed tomographic (CT) section through the temporal bone, which reveals that an axis line drawn through the ear canal ends in the attic rather than the mesotympanum. The only structure that is in the way is the scutum, and its removal allows wide and open access to the attic, which is the natural cul de sac of the external auditory canal. Rediscovering the ear canal as the access port for cholesteatoma surgery is the main story and the main advantage of endoscopic ear surgery. This approach allows more natural and direct access to and pursuit of cholesteatoma within the middle ear cleft. In contrast, traditional approaches to the attic and facial recess have provided primarily keyhole access through postauricular mastoidectomy, and many surgeons use the ear canal to access the anterior part of the attic, even during postauricular tympanomastoidectomy. Other areas, such as the hypotympanum and sinus tympani, are minimally accessible even with extensive postauricular mastoidectomy. The wide view provided by the endoscope enables minimally invasive transcanal access to all those areas and facilitates the complete extirpation of disease without the need for a postauricular approach or incision.

Transcanal Endoscopic Anatomy of the Tympanic Cavity

As discussed earlier, the transcanal endoscopic approach provides a new way of looking at the anatomy of the tympanic cavity and, more specifically, the cholesteatoma-bearing areas of that cavity. The endoscope also allows a better

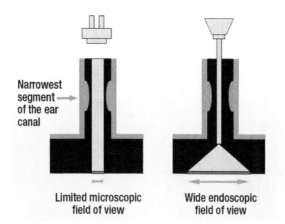

Fig. 2. The view from the microscope during transcanal surgery is defined and limited by the narrowest segment of the ear canal. In contrast, the endoscope bypasses this narrow segment and provides a wide view that allows the surgeon to look around corners, even when the 0-degree scope is used.

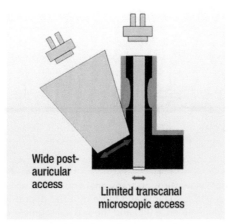

Fig. 3. The limited view provided by the microscope during transcanal procedures has forced surgeons to perform postauricular mastoidectomy, in which a port parallel to the attic is created after a considerable amount of healthy bone has been removed to enable anterior keyhole access to the attic.

understanding of the ligaments and folds of the middle ear and how they affect ventilation of these different spaces. This section highlights the anatomy of some areas and reviews the concept of the epitympanic diaphragm, which plays an important role in the pathophysiology of attic cholesteatoma.[31–33]

Facial recess

Using the transcanal endoscopic approach, the facial recess becomes an accessible and shallow depression on the posterior wall of the tympanic cavity (**Fig. 5**). In contrast, the postauricular posterior tympanotomy provides keyhole access to this important area. The pyramidal eminence, along with the vertical segment of the facial nerve, forms the medial wall of the recess and helps to mark the depth of the vertical segment of the facial nerve in that area. The bony annulus that forms the lateral wall of

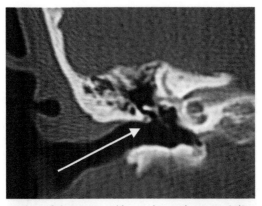

Fig. 4. A coronal CT section of the temporal bone shows that an axis line drawn through the ear canal ends in the attic rather than the mesotympanum. This almost universal anatomic orientation enables a natural transcanal access to the attic.

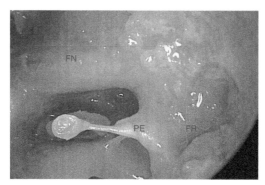

Fig. 5. Left ear. Endoscopic view through transcanal endoscopic access after minor removal of bone; the facial recess (FR) is shallow and more of a flat depression, more or less at the same level as the pyramidal eminence (PE) and the vertical segment of the facial nerve (FN).

the recess can be taken down safely as long as the pyramidal eminence is continuously observed. The relationship of the bony annulus to the vertical segment of the facial nerve is variable moving inferiorly beyond the pyramidal eminence, and great care should be taken when removing bone from the inferior/posterior aspect of the ear canal and bony annulus.

Retrotympanum When observing the anatomy of the retrotympanum, it is useful to start by identifying the footplate and the round window. The footplate is located within the posterior sinus that extends around it and posterior to it. The round window is located within the sinus subtympanicum that extends posterior and inferior to it. In between these 2 sinuses lies the sinus tympani (**Fig. 6**). It is a useful exercise during surgery to start superiorly with the posterior sinus and the footplate, and move inferiorly, identifying the ponticulus, the sinus tympani, the subiculum, and ending up with the sinus subtympanicum where the round window is located (**Fig. 7**). Inferior to that is the hypotympanum, which is separated from the sinus subtympanicum by the finiculus (**Fig. 8**).

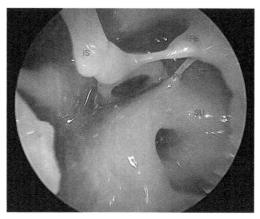

Fig. 6. Left ear: View of the retrotympanum. IS, incudostapedial joint; PE, pyramidal eminence; PO, ponticulus; RW, round window; ST, sinus tympani; SU, subiculum.

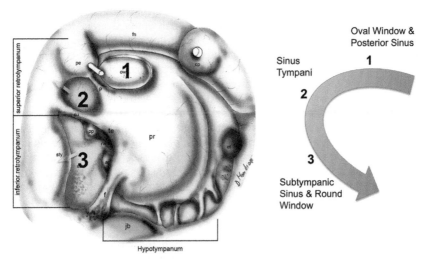

Fig. 7. The retrotympanum in a right ear. It is useful to start superiorly at the oval window and move inferiorly: from the posterior sinus, then the sinus tympani, the sinus subtympanicum, and the hypotympanum. Fn, facial nerve; jb, jugular bulb; p, ponticulus; pr, promontory; sty, styloid prominence; su, subiculum; te, temen of the round window.

Attic The attic forms a compartment that is distinct and separate from the mesotympanum both anatomically and in terms of aeration. Attic retraction pockets present often as an isolated finding with normal ventilation and findings within the mesotympanum. The concept of the epitympanic diaphragm had been advocated and advanced by many clinicians, histologists, and pathologists.[31–33] However, this concept did not make much of an inroad on the clinical side because of the difficulty in communicating and understanding the difficult anatomy. The endoscope allows a much better understanding of the anatomy of the attic and the reason that this area is distinct and separate from the rest of the middle ear in terms of ventilation.

The attic is a reasonably busy place with the bulk of the ossicular chains and many suspensory ligaments and folds. In the lateral attic, the lateral incudomallear and the

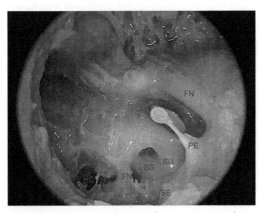

Fig. 8. Left ear: the tympanic cavity with special attention to the retrotympanum. CA, carotid artery; FN, facial nerve; FN, finiculus; HC, hypotympanic air cell; RW, round window; SE, styloid eminence; SS, sinus subtympanicus; SU, subiculum.

lateral mallear folds form a lateral wall that does not allow for ventilation of the attic via the mesotympanum laterally (**Fig. 9**). The anterior part of these lateral folds forms the medial wall of the Proussak space. The anterior attic is often separated from the anterior mesotympanum and the eustachian tubes by the tensor tympani folds. There are 2 main variations of this structure. The first is an almost horizontal orientation where the folds attach to the tensor tendon posteriorly and to the tympanic wall anteriorly close to the anterior tympanic spine (**Figs. 10** and **11**). The second is when the supratubal recess is well developed and it pushes the folds almost to a vertical position (**Fig. 12**). The attic and the supratubal recess are 2 distinct areas anatomically and developmentally. Anatomically, the supratubal recess is often a smooth-walled cavity; in contrast, the attic wall has numerous tags and excrescences. These 2 areas are separated by the transverse crest, a semicircular bony ridge that starts at the medial wall of the attic, runs across the roof, and then the lateral wall of the attic (**Fig. 13**). Its medial limb starts from the area of the cochleariform process and forms the cog, a commonly recognized surgical term, and a bony protrusion on the medial anterior attic wall (see **Fig. 13**).[34]

Developmentally, the middle ear spaces are formed from 4 pouches or sacs (saccus anticus, saccus medius, saccus superior, and saccus posticus) that bud out from the eustachian tube.[35] The attic is formed from the saccus medius, which divides into 3 saccules, anterior, medial, and posterior. The supratubal recess may be formed by the saccus anticus. The anterior saccule of the saccus medius meets the slower growing saccus anticus at the level of the semicanal of the tensor tympani, thus forming the horizontally lined tensor tympani fold. The space thus formed above the tensor fold and anterior to the tensor tendon is the anterior attic compartment.[36] Alternatively; the saccus anticus may occasionally extend upward to the tegmen, pushing the tensor fold into an almost vertical position and in the process, forming a well-developed supratubal space.[36] The expansion from the bony eustachian tube to form the supratubal recess begins at a late fetal stage and continues throughout childhood.[37] By contrast, growth of the tympanic cavity, the attic, and the mastoid antrum is virtually complete by birth.[38]

In the presence of an intact tensor fold, there is a fully formed diaphragm that separates the attic from the mesotympanum (**Fig. 14**). This diaphragm is formed by the lateral incudomallear and mallear folds laterally and the tensor folds anteriorly. The only ventilation port is through the anterior and posterior isthmus. The anterior isthmus is the area in between the incudostapedial joint and the tensor tympani tendon

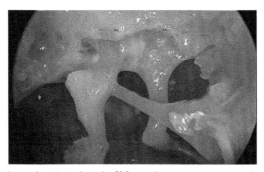

Fig. 9. Left ear: the lateral attic is closed off from the mesotympanum by the lateral incudomallear and mallear ligament. Not the relatively straight insertion line of the lateral incudomallear ligament (IML) and the downward sloping insertion line of the lateral mallear ligament (LML).

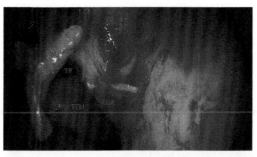

Fig. 10. Right ear: poorly developed supratubal recess in a surgical case. Using a 70° endoscope and looking up and backward. The tensor fold in these settings is almost a horizontal structure. ABA, anterior bony annulus; HM, handle of malleus; TF, tensor fold; TTM, tensor tympani muscle.

(**Fig. 15**).[32] The posterior isthmus is the area posterior to the incudostapedial joint and is often extremely narrow and has many other structures such as the chorda and the pyramidal eminence. So the anterior isthmus, or the isthmus is the main point of attic ventilation with a long channel that extends medial to the ossicles and then superior to the ossicles to ventilate the lateral and anterior attic (**Fig. 16**). This long channel is also populated by other partial folds and suspensory ligaments that provide other opportunities for impaired ventilation.

Basic Techniques and Management Algorithm

There are 3 basic approaches to the endoscopic management of cholesteatoma that echo the principles and lessons learned from traditional tympanomastoid surgical procedures. These are:

1. Transcanal management of limited cholesteatoma
2. Open endoscopic management of cholesteatoma
3. Extended transcanal approach to cholesteatoma

Although preoperative planning based on high-resolution CT and endoscopic examination is important, the decision is finally made in the operating room and patients needs to understand the range of possible interventions. The first question to be answered is whether the ear canal is an adequate port for the complete removal

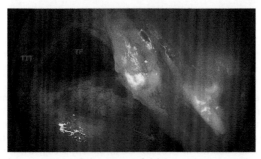

Fig. 11. Right ear: close up view of the tensor fold (*arrow*) seen in **Fig. 32**. TF, tensor fold; TTM, tensor tympani muscle bony encasement; TTT, tensor tympani tendon inserting on the neck of the malleus.

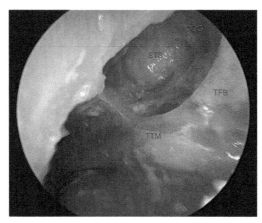

Fig. 12. Left ear: the anatomy of the tensor fold in a specimen with a well-developed supra-tubal recess. The tensor fold is composed of 2 segments, a vertical part that attaches to the cog and a horizontal part that forms a partial floor of the supratubal recess. COG, the surface of Sheehy's cogs, which separate the supratubal recess from the anterior attic; STS, supratubal recess; TFA, the vertical segment of the tensor fold, which, when complete, closes off the attic from the eustachian tube; TFB, the horizontal segment of the tensor fold that forms a partial floor of the supratubal recess anteriorly; TTM, tensor tympani muscle's bony encasement.

of cholesteatoma. If the answer is yes, then a wide tympanomeatal flap is elevated, atticotomy is performed, the sac is identified, and pursued along with removal of over-hanging bone, basically all the steps involved in the section on endoscopic management of limited cholesteatoma. If the answer is no, then the ear canal access is improved through an extended transcanal approach by removing the skin and enlarging the canal.

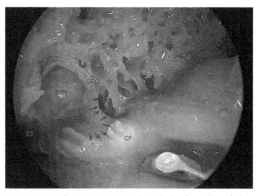

Fig. 13. Left ear: the tensor tendon is transected and the handle of the malleus is removed, as well as the anterior spine, anterior mallear ligament, and the corda tympani. Note the distinction between the smooth wall of the supratubal recess and the numerous tags and excrescences of the anterior attic. 1G, first genue of the facial nerve and neighboring genic-ulate ganglion; CG, cochleariform process; COG, Sheehy's cog; ET, eustachian tube; LC, lateral semicircular canal; STR, supratubal recess; TM, remnant tensor fold. Solid arrows, insertion point of the completely removed horizontal segment of the tensor fold; thin arrows, insertion point of the partially removed vertical segment of the tensor fold.

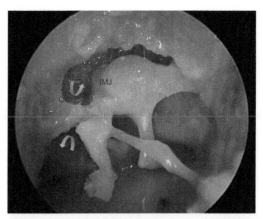

Fig. 14. Left ear: the anterior attic is separated from the supratubal recess and the eustachian tube by the tensor fold, so there is no direct communication or ventilation anteriorly between the attic and the eustachian tube.

The issue of the mastoid needs to be addressed. A limited cholesteatoma that extends to the aditus antrum can be completely removed through a transcanal approach. If the mastoid is involved, then a decision needs to be made whether the disease can be addressed through a postauricular mastoidectomy or whether it can be exteriorized by endoscopic open cavity management of cholesteatoma with aggressive bone removal superiorly and posteriorly all the way to the mastoid cavity proper (**Fig. 17**).

Endoscopic Transcanal Management of Limited Cholesteatoma

The attic (especially its anterior part) is poorly visualized via traditional approaches. An endoscopic approach enables the surgeon to retrace the sac, starting from the mesotympanum and continuing through its twists and turns around the ossicles and ligaments. This improved access also facilitates better preservation of the ossicles while

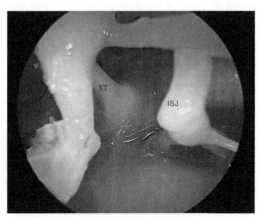

Fig. 15. Left ear: IM, the isthmus forms the only pathway for attic ventilation in the presence of a complete tensor fold. ISJ, incudostapedial joint; TT, tensor tympani tendon.

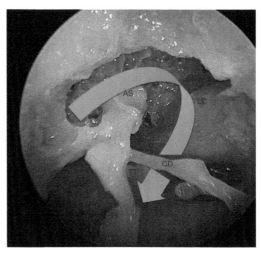

Fig. 16. Left ear: the incus has been removed to demonstrate the long narrow channel for ventilation of the attic through the isthmus, medial attic, and the upper attic.

ensuring complete removal of the matrix in toto rather than piecemeal and through different access ports.

Technique

A wide posterior tympanomeatal flap is elevated. The sac is then pursued under direct vision, and the bony rim is curetted or drilled just enough to enable dissection to continue under direct vision. Appropriate ossicular chain work is performed, and the attic defect is closed by means of a composite tragal graft.

Results

Seventy-three ear procedures were performed on 69 patients; 65 of those individuals underwent unilateral surgery. The results of preoperative CT scanning of the temporal bone, which was performed on 46 ears, suggested cholesteatoma with the presence of bony erosion in 26 ears. Seven ears showed evidence of total opacification of the middle ear and mastoid air cells (without bone erosion), and isolated opacification of the middle ear and attic was evident in 11 ears. The results of audiologic testing showed an air-bone gap of 20 dB or more in 51 ears. The transcanal endoscopic approach was adequate for the removal of disease in all patients. There were no iatrogenic facial nerve injuries. Bone thresholds were stable; ie, no change of 10 dB or more was noted in average bone conduction thresholds at 500, 1000, 2000, or 3000 Hz. In 24 ears, the cholesteatoma was dissected from the malleus head and the body of the incus, both of which were preserved. The incus or its remnant was removed in 49 ears, and the head of the malleus was removed in 43 ears. Primary ossicular reconstruction was performed in 38 ears and was delayed in 17 ears. Follow-up was performed at 43 months, on average. Revision for recurrent and clinically evident disease was performed on 5 ears. In 8 ears, a revision procedure was performed to correct a failed ossicular reconstruction or a persistent perforation. In 1 of those reconstruction failures, a small incidental pearl attached to the underlayer of the tympanic membrane was noted. Moderate-to-severe retraction in other areas of the tympanic membrane was evident in 28 patients, none of whom required further intervention.

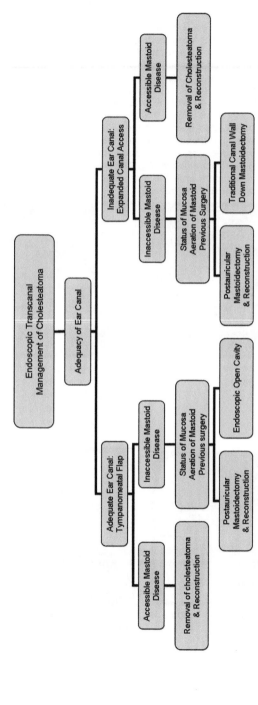

Fig. 17. The management algorithm for endoscopic transcanal management of cholesteatoma.

Case presentation: endoscopic transcanal approach

The initial evaluation of a 46-year-old man with a long-standing history of problems showed severe retraction bilaterally and some granulation tissue and drainage from the right ear. After a week of medical treatment, his right ear showed clear evidence of severe retraction and debris within the cholesteatoma sac (**Fig. 18**). An endoscopic transcanal approach was undertaken, a wide tympanomeatal flap was elevated, and the middle ear was entered (**Fig. 19**). A wide atticotomy was performed with a curette (**Fig. 20**). The cholesteatoma sac was identified; it extended to the lateral attic and was pulled downward laterally to the body of the incus and medially to the removed scutum (**Fig. 21**). Another process of the sac had rotated posteriorly and medially around the incudostapedial joint and the superstructure of the stapes and had advanced medially to the long process of the incus (**Fig. 22**). The sac was pulled out completely and was deflected (**Fig. 23**). It was evident that the sac had eroded the incudostapedial joint (**Fig. 24**). A prosthesis was used to reconstruct the ossicular chain (**Fig. 25**). A piece of tragal composite graft with excess perichondrium was used to reconstruct the attic defect (**Fig. 26**). The tympanic membrane defect was reconstructed with a perichondrial underlay graft, and the tympanomeatal flap was repositioned (**Fig. 27**). The patient experienced an uneventful postoperative course. One month after the procedure, his tympanic membrane was intact, his hearing was good, and he returned to duty.

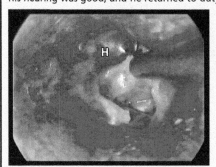

Fig. 18. Right ear: note the retraction and cholesteatoma. H, handle of malleus.

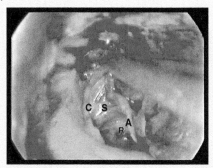

Fig. 19. Right ear: the tympanomeatal flap has been elevated, the middle ear has been entered, and the cholesteatoma sac has been exposed. A, annulus; C, chorda tympani; R, round window; S, cholesteatoma sac.

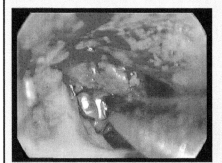

Fig. 20. Right ear: a wide atticotomy is performed with a curette.

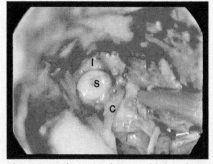

Fig. 21. Right ear: the sac (S) has been pulled down from the attic, lateral to the body of the incus, and medial to the scutum. The body of the incus (I) can be seen. The chorda (C) forms a collar around the neck of the sac.

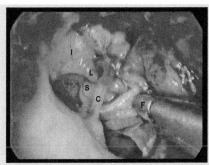

Fig. 22. Right ear: the sac has been completely pulled down from the area lateral to the body of the incus (I), but another process of the sac (S) has rotated posteriorly and medially around the incudostapedial joint and medial to the long process of the incus (L). Cuffed forceps (F) are used to pull the sac from underneath the chorda (C).

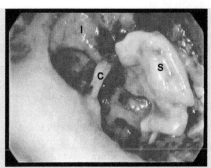

Fig. 23. Right ear: The sac (S) has been completely pulled out and deflected over the tympanomeatal flap with the incus (I) and the chorda (C) in view.

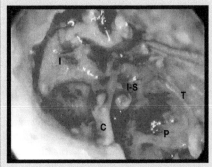

Fig. 24. Right ear: the sac is removed. The cholesteatoma has eroded the incudostapedial joint (I-S). The incus (I), the chorda (C), and the promontory (P) are clearly in view. The anterior edge of the tympanic membrane retraction (T), now a perforation, is also visible.

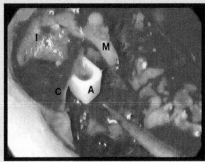

Fig. 25. Right ear: a prosthesis (A) is used to reconstruct the incudostapedial joint. The handle of the malleus (M), the incus (I), and chorda (C) are visible.

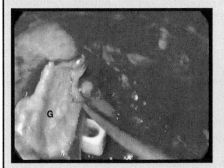

Fig. 26. Right ear: the attic defect is reconstructed by means of a composite tragal graft (G) with excess perichondrium to prevent retraction around the graft.

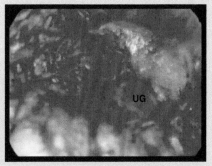

Fig. 27. Right ear: the tympanomeatal flap is repositioned over an underlay graft (UG) to reconstruct the retracted area of the tympanic membrane.

Endoscopic Open Cavity Management of Cholesteatoma

In canal wall down procedures, which have been viewed as the definitive treatment of cholesteatoma, all disease-containing cavities are exteriorized to provide natural aeration and direct access to the disease in the clinic setting. However, during the process of accessing the disease, large problematic cavities that require lifelong maintenance are created. In addition, unpredictable healing patterns, fibrosis, and closing of the meatus, which are common complications associated with postauricular canal wall down procedures, often prevent further ossicular reconstruction. Endoscopic techniques allow transcanal exploration of the disease-containing cavities without opening up areas that are not involved in the cholesteatoma. Such techniques enable the surgeon to approach and reconstruct the ear in a highly predictable fashion. This in turn creates a better framework for ossicular and partial tympanic membrane reconstruction.

The transcanal endoscopic approach opens up only diseased areas, preserves many healthy air cells, and leaves the cortical bone intact. It also allows for the creation of 2 independent cavities: the small reconstructed tympanic cavity that conducts sound in the middle ear and is small enough to be serviced by the usually dysfunctional eustachian tube, and the larger attic, antrum, and mastoid cavities, which are joined to the ear canal and are exteriorized (**Fig. 28**). Such an approach was described by Tos[27] in 1982. The main concern of many surgeons is the possibility of closing the open attic. That concern is driven by the results of traditional open surgery of the mastoid, in which damage to the cartilaginous portion of the ear canal produces a vicious circle: Trauma to the ear canal results in fibrosis and narrowing of the meatus, which forces the surgeon to design a more aggressive meatoplasty, which in turn results in more trauma, secondary fibrosis, and narrowing. A huge meatus must be created to compensate for that eventual fibrosis and narrowing. In contrast, the limited trauma to the cartilaginous ear canal caused by endoscopic surgery allows surgeons to avoid those complications and results in small, shallow, benign, problem-free cavities.

Technique

In endoscopic open cavity management of cholesteatoma, the wide posterior tympanomeatal flap is elevated as described earlier. A transcanal atticotomy is performed. The attic is then emptied from the incus and the head of the malleus. Aggressive bone removal is then performed to provide open endoscopic access into the attic and all the way posteriorly into the antrum. Tympanic membrane defects inferior to the horizontal segment of the facial nerve (including atelectatic areas) are

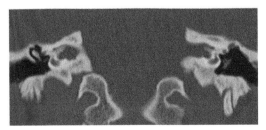

Fig. 28. Coronal CT views of a patient who underwent endoscopic open cavity management of a cholesteatoma in the left ear. Compare the normal ear to the left operated ear. The neotympanic membrane (NT) is reconstructed up to the level of the horizontal segment of the facial nerve (FN), and the attic is left open (OA).

Case presentation: endoscopic open cavity management of cholesteatoma

The patient was 41 years old with a retraction pocket and recurrent granulation tissue. **Fig. 29** shows the large attic retraction pocket after it was emptied of dermal debris. A wide tympanomeatal flap was elevated, and the thick vascularized sac can be seen after the atticotomy was extended (**Figs. 30 and 31**). The incus and the head of the malleus were removed after the incudostapedial joint was dislocated (**Figs. 32 and 33**). The anterior epitympanum was cleared of all disease. The remainder of the sac deep to the removed ossicles was removed after further widening of the atticotomy (**Fig. 34**). All disease was excised, and specific attention was paid to the attic and the tympanic cavity (**Fig. 35**). A prosthesis was used to reconstruct the ossicular chain (**Fig. 36**), and a composite cartilage graft was positioned on top of the prosthesis (**Fig. 37**). The tympanomeatal flap was divided longitudinally (**Fig. 38**). The inferior part was repositioned over the ear canal, the superior part was draped over the horizontal segment of the facial nerve (**Fig. 39**), and the attic was packed open.

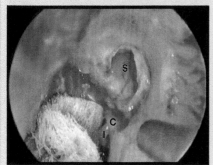

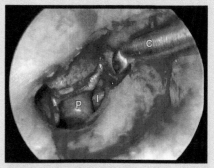

Fig. 29. Left ear: a large retraction pocket (RP) with evidence of recurrent prior episodes of infections and the formation of granulation tissue. HM, handle of malleus; TM, tympanic membrane.

Fig. 30. Left ear: a wide tympanomeatal flap is elevated. The premonitory (P) and the incudostapedial joint (I) can be seen. A curette is used (C) to create the extended atticotomy.

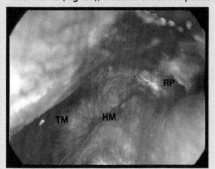

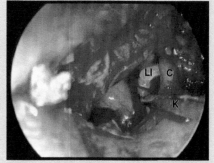

Fig. 31. Left ear: note the extended atticotomy at the thick sac (S), the chorda tympani (C), and the incudostapedial joint (I).

Fig. 32. Left ear: the incudostapedial joint (LI) is dislocated with a small round knife (K). C, chorda tympani.

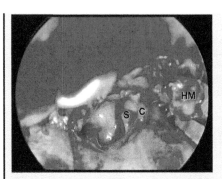

Fig. 33. Left ear: the incus has been removed, and the head of the malleus (HM) is extracted. Note that the head of the malleus is separated from the handle by means of a malleus nipper at a proximal site to preserve the ligaments stabilizing the handle of malleus. C, chorda tympani; S, stapes.

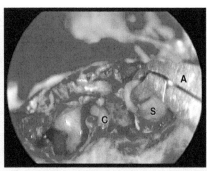

Fig. 34. Left ear: the thick sac (S) is being pulled with an alligator forceps (A). C, chorda tympani.

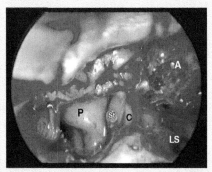

Fig. 35. Left ear: the sac has been removed completely. A, attic; C, chorda tympani; LS, lateral semicircular canal; P, promontory; S, stapes.

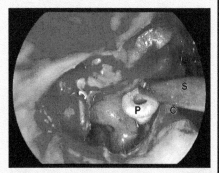

Fig. 36. The ossicular chain is reconstructed with the use of a prosthesis (P). C, chorda tympani; S, suction.

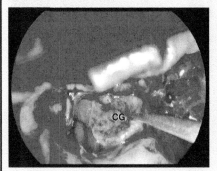

Fig. 37. Left ear: composite tragal cartilage (CG) is used on top of the prosthesis.

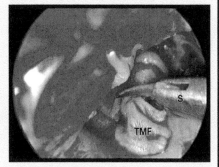

Fig. 38. Left ear: the tympanomeatal flap is cut longitudinally with middle ear scissors.

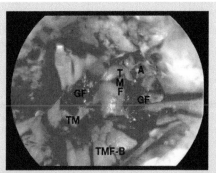

Fig. 39. Left ear: the inferior part of the tympanomeatal flap (TMF-B) is repositioned over the ear canal while the superior part of the tympanomeatal flap (TMF) is reflected over the horizontal segment of the facial nerve into the open attic (A). Small pieces of Gelfoam (GF) are used to pack the open attic and ear canal. TM, tympanic membrane.

reconstructed with a perichondrial graft, which is placed directly on, and up to, the horizontal segment of the facial nerve superiorly and on a bed of Gelfoam that is packed in the middle ear inferiorly. The ear canal and the open attic are then packed with Gelfoam. This technique should result in a small, closed, reconstructed tympanic cavity and membrane anteriorly and inferiorly (to service the impedance-matching function of the middle ear) and an open attic and antrum posteriorly and superiorly (see **Fig. 28**).

Results
Eighty-five ear procedures were performed on 78 patients. There were no iatrogenic facial nerve injuries. Bone thresholds were stable (stability was defined as no change of 10 dB or more in average bone conduction thresholds at 500, 1000, 2000, and 3000 Hz) except in 1 patient who presented preoperatively with depressed bone thresholds, vertigo, and a perilymphatic fistula. The mean follow-up was 32 months. Closure of the air-bone gap to within 20 dB was accomplished in 47 ears. Six ears required revision

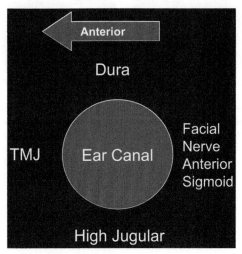

Fig. 40. Structures to be considered when enlarging the ear canal. TMJ, tympanomeatal flap.

Case presentation: expanded transcanal access to the middle ear and petrous apex

A 36-year-old man presented with a long-standing history of right hearing loss and dizziness. Examination showed an anterior whitish lesion behind the tympanic membrane (**Fig. 41**). Audiometry indicated a dead ear on the right, normal hearing on the left. CT of the temporal bone showed extensive petrous bone cholesteatoma eroding the cochlea and the carotid artery (**Fig. 42**). Using the expanded transcanal access technique, the vascular strip was preserved, the ear canal skin was removed, the fibrous layer of the tympanic membrane was preserved, and the ear canal was then enlarged (**Fig. 43**). The extensive cholesteatoma had eroded the bony encasement of the sinus tympani muscle and carotid and had eroded the middle and apical turns of the cochlea (**Fig. 44**). The cholesteatoma was completely removed from the apex of the petrous bone (**Fig. 45**).

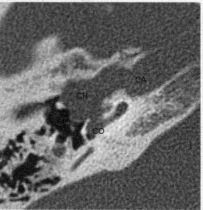

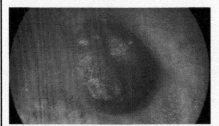

Fig. 41. Right ear with an anterior whitish lesion behind an intact tympanic membrane.

Fig. 42. Right ear: axial CT images of the temporal bone. CO, basal turn of the cochlea; CA, carotid artery; CH, cholesteatoma.

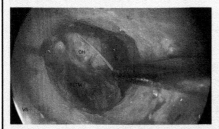

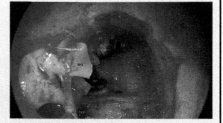

Fig. 43. Right ear: the skin of the ear canal is elevated in contiguity with the epithelial layer of the tympanic membrane with preservation of the vascular strip and then enlargement of ear canal. CH, cholesteatoma; FLTM, fibrous layer of tympanic membrane; VS, vascular strip.

Fig. 44. Right ear: much of the cholesteatoma eroding the cochlea has been removed. CA, eroded carotid artery canal; CH, cholesteatoma in the petrous apex surrounding the tensor tympani muscle (TT); CO, the eroded middle turn of the cochlea; MAL, malleus with the handle transected; SFP, stapes footplate.

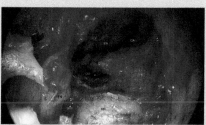

Fig. 45. Right ear: the view after complete removal of a cholesteatoma. CA, carotid artery; CO, eroded middle turn of cochlea; FN, dehiscent facial nerve; PA, petrous apex; PR, promontory; SFP, stapes footplate.

surgery, Four of the surgical failures resulted from complete closure of the open attic by a growth of overlying skin rather than by a step-by-step narrowing of the atticotomy. This complication was usually evident early in the postoperative course and was managed by re-excising the overlying skin in a simple procedure.

Expanded Transcanal Access to the Middle Ear and Petrous Apex

Although the use of the endoscope allows much expanded transcanal access to the middle ear compared with the microscope, the ear canal in some patients can be so limiting in size and angulation that adequate exposure is not possible. Addressing these limitations before addressing the disease is essential for performing adequate and safe endoscopic procedures. In addition, this approach provides wide access to disease within the anterior middle ear, eustachian tube, and the petrous bone.

Technique

After evaluation of the limiting elements in the ear canal in relation to location of the disease, a decision is made on whether to address these limitations. The location of disease and its extent is determined by endoscopic examination and review of CT of the temporal bone. Anterior middle ear, eustachian tube, and significant disease within the hypotympanum often require an expanded transcanal approach. When enlarging the ear canal, the surgeon needs to be keenly aware of critical structures that lie in close proximity (**Fig. 40**). The bony annulus, the line separating the ear canal from the middle ear, has tremendous variations[39] and all the structures that border the tympanic cavity proper should be considered when enlarging the ear canal. Posteriorly, the facial nerve and an anterior sigmoid should be condsidered.[40] Inferiorly, a high jugular bulb can come lateral to and border the ear canal.[41] Breaching the glenoid fossa anteriorly is usually a nonevent, but it can present a limiting factor.

The technique echoes that of Sheehy's lateral graft tympanoplasty. The skin of the ear canal is removed along with the epithelial layer of the tympanic membrane and the vascular strip is preserved. The ear canal is enlarged as needed. The annulus and the fibrous layer of the tympanic membrane are elevated either completely or partially to provide access to the areas of interest. Then all of the overhanging bony annulus is curetted and wide access to the middle ear is gained for removal of any disease. After the necessary ossicular chain work, the remaining part of the tympanic membrane is repositioned, a lateral graft is applied, and the skin of the ear canal is repositioned and packed in place.

SUMMARY

The story of endoscopic management of cholesteatoma is that of the rediscovering the ear canal as the most logical, direct, and natural access point to cholesteatoma within the mesotympanum, attic, facial recess, sinus tympany, hpotympanum, and eustachian tube. It offers a fresh outlook on this disease and changes the surgical treatment paradigm of cholesteatoma.

SUPPLEMENTARY DATA

Supplementary data related to this article can be found online at http://dx.doi.org/10.1016/j.otc.2012.10.001.

REFERENCES

1. Thomassin JM, Korchia D, Doris JM. Endoscopic-guided otosurgery in the prevention of residual cholesteatomas. Laryngoscope 1993;103:939–43.
2. Hawke M. Telescopic otoscopy and photography of the tympanic membrane. J Otolaryngol 1982;11:35–9.
3. Nomura Y. Effective photography in otolaryngology-head and neck surgery: endoscopic photography of the middle ear. Otolaryngol Head Neck Surg 1982; 90:395–8.
4. Takahashi H, Honjo I, Fujita A, et al. Transtympanic endoscopic findings in patients with otitis media with effusion. Arch Otolaryngol Head Neck Surg 1990;116: 1186–9.
5. Poe DS, Bottrill ID. Comparison of endoscopic and surgical explorations for perilymphatic fistulas. Am J Otol 1994;15:735–8.
6. McKennan KX. Endoscopic 'second look' mastoidoscopy to rule out residual epitympanic/mastoid cholesteatoma. Laryngoscope 1993;103:810–4.
7. Tarabichi M. Endoscopic management of acquired cholesteatoma. Am J Otol 1997;18:544–9.
8. Tarabichi M. Endoscopic middle ear surgery. Ann Otol Rhinol Laryngol 1999;108: 39–46.
9. Tarabichi M. Endoscopic management of cholesteatoma: long-term results. Otolaryngol Head Neck Surg 2000;122:874–81.
10. Tarabichi M. Endoscopic management of limited attic cholesteatoma. Laryngoscope 2004;114:1157–62.
11. Kakehata S, Futai K, Sasaki A, et al. Endoscopic transtympanic tympanoplasty in the treatment of conductive hearing loss: early results. Otol Neurotol 2006;27(1): 14–9.
12. Kakehata S, Hozawa K, Futai K, et al. Evaluation of attic retraction pockets by microendoscopy. Otol Neurotol 2005;26(5):834–7.
13. Kakehata S, Futai K, Kuroda R, et al. Office-based endoscopic procedure for diagnosis in conductive hearing loss cases using OtoScan Laser-Assisted Myringotomy. Laryngoscope 2004;114(7):1285–9.
14. Badr-el-Dine M. Value of ear endoscopy in cholesteatoma surgery. Otol Neurotol 2002;23:631–5.
15. El-Meselaty K, Badr-El-Dine M, Mandour M, et al. Endoscope affects decision making in cholesteatoma surgery. Otolaryngol Head Neck Surg 2003;129:490–6.
16. Yung MW. The use of middle ear endoscopy: has residual cholesteatoma been eliminated? J Laryngol Otol 2001;115:958–61.

17. Ayache S, Tramier B, Strunski V. Otoendoscopy in cholesteatoma surgery of the middle ear. What benefits can be expected? Otol Neurotol 2008;29(8):1085–90.
18. Abdel Baki F, Badr-El-Dine M, El Saiid I, et al. Sinus tympani endoscopic anatomy. Otolaryngol Head Neck Surg 2002;127:158–62.
19. Mattox DE. Endoscopy-assisted surgery of the petrous apex. Otolaryngol Head Neck Surg 2004;130:229–41.
20. Magnan J, Sanna M. Endoscopy in neuro-otology. Stuttgart (Germany): Georg Thieme Verlag; 2003.
21. Badr-El-Dine M, El-Garem HF, Talaat AM, et al. Endoscopically assisted minimally invasive microvascular decompression of hemifacial spasm. Otol Neurotol 2002; 23:122–8.
22. El-Garem HF, Badr-El-Dine M, Talaat AM, et al. Endoscopy as a tool in minimally invasive trigeminal neuralgia surgery. Otol Neurotol 2002;23:132–5.
23. Badr-El-Dine M, El-Garem HF, El-Ashram Y, et al. Endoscope assisted minimal invasive microvascular decompression of hemifacial spasm. Abstracts of the 9th International Facial Nerve Symposium. Otol Neurotol 2002;23(Suppl 3): 68–72.
24. Rosenberg SI, Silverstein H, Willcox TO, et al. Endoscopy in otology and neuro-tology. Am J Otol 1994;15:168–72.
25. Presutti L, Marchioni D, Mattioli F, et al. Endoscopic management of acquired cholesteatoma: our experience. Otolaryngol Head Neck Surg 2008;37(4):1–7.
26. Marchioni D, Mattioli F, Ciufelli MA, et al. Endoscopic approach to tensor fold in patients with attic cholesteatoma. Acta Otolaryngol 2008;19:1–9.
27. Tos M. Modification of combined-approach tympanoplasty in attic cholesteatoma. Arch Otolaryngol 1982;108:772–8.
28. Sheehy JL, Brackmann DE, Graham MD. Cholesteatoma surgery: residual and recurrent disease. A review of 1,024 cases. Ann Otol Rhinol Laryngol 1977;86:451–62.
29. Glasscock ME, Miller GW. Intact canal wall tympanoplasty in the management of cholesteatoma. Laryngoscope 1976;86:1639–57.
30. Kinney SE. Five years experience using the intact canal wall tympanoplasty with mastoidectomy for cholesteatoma: preliminary report. Laryngoscope 1982;92: 1395–400.
31. Chatellier HP, Lemoine J. Le diaphragme interattico-tympanique du 612 nouveau-né. Description de sa morphologie considérations sur son role 613 pathogénique dans les otomastoidites cloisonnées du nourisson. Ann 614 Otolaryngol Chir Cervicofac (Paris) 1945;13:534–66 [in French].
32. Aimi K. The tympanic isthmus: its anatomy and clinical significance. Laryngoscope 1978;88(7 Pt 1):1067–81.
33. Palva T, Ramsay H. Incudal folds and epitympanic aeration. Am J Otol 1996;17: 700–8.
34. Palva T, Ramsay H, Böhling T. Tensor fold and anterior epitympanum. Am J Otol 1997;18:307–16.
35. Hammar JA. Studien Über Die Entwicklung Des Vorderdarms und Einiger Angrenzenden Organe. Arch Mikroskop Anat 1902;59:471–628 [in German].
36. Proctor B. The development of the middle ear spaces and their surgical significance. J Laryngol Otol 1964;78:631–48.
37. Tono T, Schachern PA, Morizono T, et al. Developmental anatomy of the supratubal recess in temporal bones from fetuses and children. Am J Otol 1996;17: 99–107.
38. Schuknecht HF, Gulya AJ. Anatomy of the temporal bone with surgical implications. Philadelphia: Lea & Febiger; 1986. p. 89–90.

39. Adad B, Rasgon BM, Ackerson L. Relationship of the facial nerve to the tympanic annulus: a direct anatomic examination. Laryngoscope 1999;109:1189–92.
40. Gangopadhyay KP, McArthur D, Larsson SG. Unusual anterior course of the sigmoid sinus: report of a case and review of the literature. J Laryngol Otol 1996;110:984–6.
41. Moore PJ. The high jugular bulb in ear surgery: three case reports and a review of the literature. J Laryngol Otol 1994;108:772–5.

Endoscopic Transcanal Ear Anatomy and Dissection

Muaaz Tarabichi, MD[a],*, Daniele Marchioni, MD[b],
Livio Presutti, MD[b], João Flávio Nogueira, MD[c], Dave Pothier, MD[d]

KEYWORDS

- Ear anatomy • Middle ear • Transcanal • Endoscopy • Cholesteatoma
- Tympanoplasty

KEY POINTS

- The endoscope allows detailed observation of the anatomy of the tympanic cavity.
- The anatomy of the ear canal is important as the access point to the tympanic.
- The Epitympanic Diaphragm separates the air containing spaces of the temporal bone into two cavities: a posterior superior mastoid/attic cavity and an anterior inferior mesotympanic/eustachian tube cavity.
- There are other mucosal folds that segment the air cavities and prevent pan ventilation of these spaces.

ENDOSCOPIC DISSECTION OF THE MIDDLE EAR

Objectives

1. Develop an understanding of the endoscopic anatomy of the middle and inner ear through transcanal access.
2. Develop the necessary hand-eye coordination and hands skills to perform endoscopic ear surgery.
3. In the laboratory, perform the specific steps involved in tympanoplasty.
4. Understand the anatomy of the cholesteatoma-bearing areas of the middle ear.
5. In the laboratory, perform the exploration of all the cholesteatoma-bearing areas of the middle ear.

A version of this article appeared in Tarabichi M, Marchioni D, Presutti L, et al. Endoscopic Transcanal Ear Anatomy and Dissection. Tuttlingen, Germany: Endo Press, 2011. Used with permission of Karl Storz GmbH & Co.
[a] Center for Ear Endoscopy, 3535 30th Avenue, Kenosha, Wisconsin, WI 53144, USA; [b] Department of Otolaryngology, University Hospital of Modena, Italy; [c] Department of Otolaryngology, Hospital Geral de Fortaleza, Fortaleza, Brazil; [d] Department of Otolaryngology-Head and Neck Surgery, University of Toronto, Toronto, Ontario, Canada
* Corresponding author.
E-mail address: tarabichi@yahoo.com

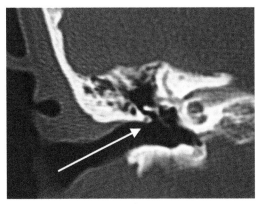

Fig. 1. Right ear: Coronal computed tomography section through the right ear canal and middle ear. Note that the axis of the ear canal slopes upward. The scutum represents the real bottom of the ear canal rather than the mesotympanum. If the scutum is removed, this would allow direct access to the attic, the area most involved in cholesteatoma. The *arrow* represents Axis of the ear canal.

Workstation and Setup

The head/temporal bone holder should be positioned in such a way that would align the axis of the ear canal with the axis of the surgeon's vision. Given the up-sloping orientation of the ear canal (**Fig. 1**), this would result in the surgeon's field of view being centered on the lateral short process of the malleus rather than the umbo of the tympanic membrane (TM). The anatomic specimen should be positioned between the monitor and the surgeon. When using the 0° endoscope and during much of the dissection, the specimen's top should be to your right for the right ear and to your left for the left ear. When using angled scopes, you should always be able to rotate the anatomic specimen around as you explore the different middle ear space. The orientation of the angled view of the endoscope should always face away from the surgeon and face the monitor.

Required Instruments

Description

- Round knife 45°, 16 cm, diameter: 2.5 mm
- Plester knife, round, vertical, 16 cm, standard size 3.5 × 2.5 mm
- Serrated Alligator forceps
- Wullstein needle, 16.5 cm, light curve
- Bellucci scissors, working length 8 cm, delicate, curved right
- Bellucci scissors, working length 8 cm, delicate, curved left
- House-Dieter malleus nipper, working length 8 cm, up biting
- House curette, 15 cm, large size
- Fisch adaptor, with cutoff hole, Luer cone 5.5 cm
- Suction cannula, angular, Luer-Lock, working length 6 cm, outer diameter (OD) 1.5 mm
- 3 mm 14 cm, 0° Hopkins telescope
- 3 mm 14 cm, 30° Hopkins telescope

Dissection Tasks

1. Inspect the ear canal
2. Outline vascular strip
3. Remove the canal skin along with the epithelial layer of TM
4. Enlarge the ear canal
5. Elevate annulus
6. Separate tympanic membrane remnant
7. Take down bony annulus
8. Enlarge access to inferior retrotympanum and hypotympanum
9. Start with a careful limited atticotomy
10. Continue and extend atticotomy
11. Remove entire scutum
12. Extend the bone removal anteriorly
13. View the articular surface, then proceed with disarticulation from the stapes and the malleus and removal of the incus
14. Transect the neck of the malleus
15. Transect the tensor tympani tendon and remove the handle of malleus

Elective task

16. Try to remove the bony encasement of the facial nerve

Dissection Tasks

Dissection Task 1: Inspection of the ear canal

It is important to spend a few minutes inspecting the anatomy of the ear canal, the TM, and whatever is visible through the transparent TM.

Observe

i. Many of the vessels of the TM run down from the ear canal, and they supply the TM from laterally to medially; this is very apparent living patients but might not be obvious in an anatomic specimen. So, by removing the skin of the canal and the epithelial layer of the TM, you have largely eliminated the bleeding elements of the external ear and TM (**Fig. 2**).

ii. The axis of the ear canal is angled superiorly and the scutum lies at the bottom of the canal (see **Fig. 1**).

iii. Observe the location and extent of any anterior overhang. Also, please note that in many specimens there is also an inferior overhang (**Fig. 3**).

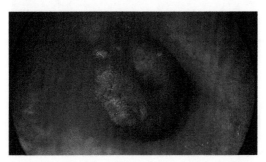

Fig. 2. Right ear: Endoscopic view of the TM in a right ear with cholesteatoma visible behind the TM. Note the blood vessels arising from the ear canal and supplying the TM.

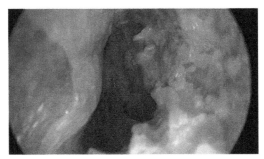

Fig. 3. Left ear: The view through the endoscope of an anatomic specimen with a small perforation. Note the size and location of the significant anterior overhang.

Dissection Task 2: Outline vascular strip

Use the round knife to make the medial cut just 2 to 3 mm away from the annulus and then use the Plester flap knife to extend the cuts laterally.

Observe

i. The fibrous annulus of the TM almost disappears in the upper posterior part of the TM (see **Fig. 2**; **Fig. 4**).
ii. You need to palpate the bony edge of the middle ear before you make your deep cut. It is usually the fibrous annulus that is visible. The lack of the fibrous annulus superiorly and the injection of the ear canal with lidocaine (Xylocaine) and epinephrine would result in an engorged vascular strip and a lack of definition of the bony annulus rim separating the ear canal from the middle ear

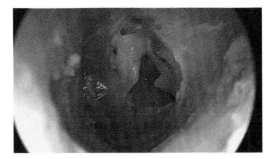

Fig. 4. Left ear: The skin of the canal has been removed along with the epithelial layer of the TM. The ear canal has been enlarged. Note the limits of the fibrous annulus (*red circles*); CT, chorda tympani; PML, posterior mallear ligament.

Dissection Task 3: Removal of the canal skin along with the epithelial layer of TM

Using the round knife, a circular lateral incision is made that connects the two limbs of the vascular strip incision across the anterior canal in preparation for the removal of the ear canal skin. Please note that the incision needs to be lateral enough to any anterior bony overhang. Then the skin of the ear canal should be elevated under direct vision. All overhanging bone is curetted away as we proceed medially in the canal. Care should be taken to avoid the temporomandibular joint. As the annulus is reached, it should not be elevated; the skin of the canal should be elevated in contiguity with the epithelial layer of the TM. This procedure is done either by running the round knife over and in the direction of the annulus inferiorly or by using a cuffed forceps to pull down the epithelial layer off of the lateral short process of the malleus superiorly. Attention should be paid to maintaining the fibrous annulus tethered to its bony groove.

Observe

i. The glistening white annulus and fibrous layer of the TM (see **Fig. 4**)
ii. The friable skin and epithelial layer of the TM (compare **Figs. 3** and **4**)

Dissection Task 4: Enlarging the ear canal

The ear canal should be curetted out in all directions to maintain a full and simultaneous view of the annulus and the ear canal with a 0° scope. Given the fact that the bony annulus separating the middle ear from the ear canal is very variable in relationship to other structures, you need to consider the possibility of a low dura, anterior sigmoid, facial nerve, and a high jugular bulb as you enlarge the ear canal (**Figs. 5** and **6**).

Dissection Task 5: Elevation of the annulus up to 1 and 6 o'clock

Using the cuffed forceps, pull down the fibrous layer of the TM off of the upper part of the handle of malleus and out of the groove of the bony annulus and deflect the elevated TM anteriorly.

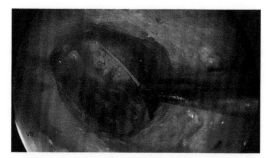

Fig. 5. Right ear: The canal wall is curetted to obtain a full view of the tympanic ring in one view using the 0° endoscope. CH, cholesteatoma; FLTM, fibrous layer of tympanic membrane; VS, vascular strip.

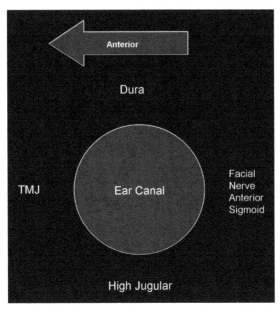

Fig. 6. The left ear canal with the surrounding structures that need to be considered when enlarging the ear canal.

Observe

i. The posterior mallear ligament overlying the chorda tympani and almost parallel to it (**Fig. 7**)
ii. The undersurface the TM and the handle of the malleus

Dissection Task 6: Separate tympanic membrane

Using a Wullstein needle, the TM remnant is separated from the handle of malleus from the lateral short process of the malleus and downward toward the umbo. Then using angled Bellucci scissors, the TM remnant is separated from the umbo (**Fig. 8**).

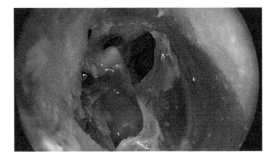

Fig. 7. Right ear: Fibrous layer of the TM is pulled down off of the handle of malleus revealing the posterior mallear ligament (PML) and the chorda tympani (CT). TMJ, tempromandibular joint.

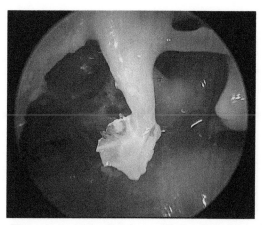

Fig. 8. Left ear: The fibrous layer of the TM along with the fibrous annulus is removed and separated from the handle of malleus. TT, the tendon of the tensor tympani.

Dissection Task 7: Take down the bony annulus posteriorly to gain full access to the facial recess and sinus tympani

Make sure that the posterior canal wall is almost flush with the pyramidal process (**Fig. 9**).

Observe

i. Using a 0° scope, the facial recess is very accessible and forms a small depression on the posterior wall of the tympanic cavity (see **Fig. 9**).

ii. Using the 30° scope, position the specimen so that the posterior aspect is away from you and orient the angle of the endoscope to look away from you. Inspect the retrotympanic anatomy (**Fig. 10**).

iii. Observe the pyramidal eminence and look for possible subpyramidal space (**Fig. 11**).

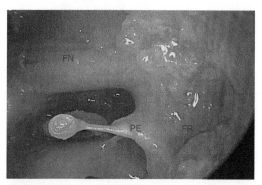

Fig. 9. Left ear: Using transcanal endoscopic access and after removal of some bone, the facial recess seems to be less of a recess and more of a slight depression just superficial to the pyramidal eminence and the vertical segment of facial nerve. FN, facial nerve; FR, facial recess; PE, pyramidal eminence.

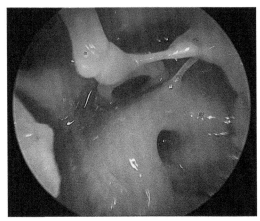

Fig. 10. Left ear: View of the retrotympanum. IS, incudostapedial joint; PE, pyramidal eminence; PO, ponticulus; RW, round window; ST, sinus tympani; SU, subiculum.

   iv. Observe the entry point for any subpyramidal space. Study the different possible variations (**Fig. 12**); inspect your specimen and compare it with the other specimens being dissected. Note that in the specimen being dissected here, it is an extension of both the sinus tympani and the posterior tympanic sinus (**Fig. 13**).
   v. Study the possible different variations in the shape of the sinus tympani (**Fig. 14**).

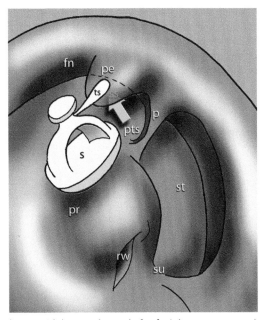

Fig. 11. Left ear: Subpyramidal space (*arrow*). fn, facial nerve; p, ponticulus; pe, pyramidal eminence; pr, promonitory; pts, posterior tympanic sinus; rw, round window; S, stapes; ss, subpyramidal space; st, sinus tympani; su, subiculum; ts, stapedius muscle tendon.

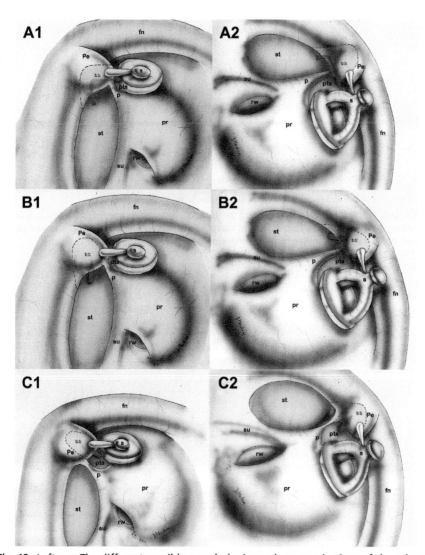

Fig. 12. Left ear: The different possible morphologies and communications of the subpyramidal space with surrounding structures. (*A1, A2*) Different perspectives of a subpyramidal space that communicates with both the posterior sinus and the sinus tympani. (*B1, B2*) Different perspectives of a subpyramidal space that is really an extension of the sinus tympani. (*C1, C2*) Different perspectives of a subpyramidal space that is really an extension of the posterior sinus. *Red Arrow,* the subpyramidal space is formed by expansion of pneumatiztion of the either the sinus tympani or the posterior sinus. fn, facial nerve; Pe, pyramidal eminence; pr, promonitory; pts, posterior tympanic sinus; rw, round window; ss, subpyramidal space; st, sinus tympani; su, subiculum.

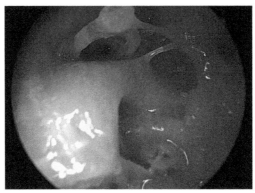

Fig. 13. Left ear: Note the entry points of the subpyramidal space in this specimen is type A, connecting to both the sinus tympani and the posterior tympanic sinus. Subpyramidal space (*arrow*). PE, pyramidal eminence; PTS, posterior tympanic sinus; ST, sinus tympani.

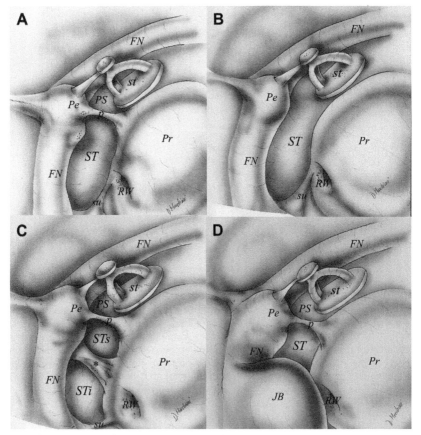

Fig. 14. The possible different morphologies of the sinus tympani. Ridge separating the sinus tympani into 2 parts (*asterisk*). FN, facial nerve; JB, jugular bulb; P, ponticulus; Pe, pyramidal eminance; Pr, prominotory; PS, posterior sinus; RW, round window; st, stapes; ST, sinus tympani; STi, inferior sinus tympani; STs, superior part of sinus tympani; su, subiculum.

vi. Study the classification of the depth of the of the sinus tympani (**Figs. 15** and **16**).

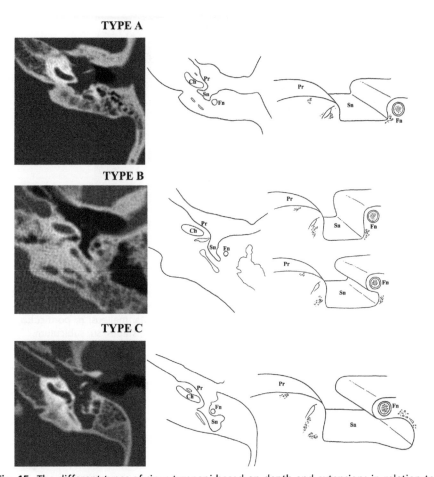

Fig. 15. The different types of sinus tympani based on depth and extensions in relation to the facial nerve. Ch, cochlea; Fn, facial nerve; Pr, promonitory; Sn, sinus tympani.

vii. Observe the shape and depth of the sinus tympani in your specimen. Try to classify (with palpation if necessary) the type of sinus tympani in your specimen (see **Fig. 10**).

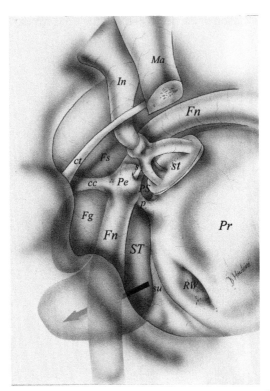

Fig. 16. Type C sinus tympani. Black arrow indicates posterior extension of ST with respect to the third portion of the facial nerve. cc, chordal ridge; ct, chorda tympani nerve; Fg, lateral tympanic sinus; Fn, facial nerve; Fs, facial sinus; In, incus; Ma, malleus; p, ponticulus; Pe, pyramidal process; PS, posterior sinus; s, stapedial tendon; ST, stapes; su, subiculum.

viii. Observe the ponticulus and its possible variations (**Fig. 17**).

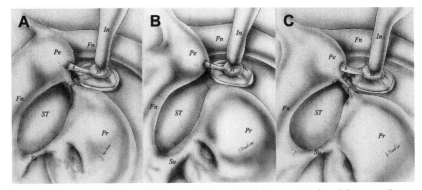

Fig. 17. Different morphology of the ponticulus. (*A*) Ridge ponticulus, (*B*) incomplete ponticulus, and (*C*) bridge ponticulus. Fn, facial nerve; In, incus; p, ponticulus; Pe, pyramidal process; Pr, prominotory; PS, posterior sinus, s, stapedial tendon; ST, stapes; Su, subiculum.

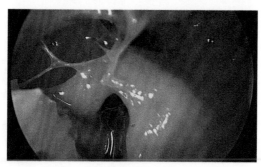

Fig. 18. Right ear round window niche. Round window membrane (*arrows*). AP, anterior pillar; PP, posterior pillar; TE, tegmen.

ix. Try to inspect the round window membrane and niche. Identify the tegmen of the round window niche and the anterior and posterior pillars (**Fig. 18**).

Dissection Task 8: Take down any inferior overhang and enlarge the access to the inferior retrotympanum and hypotympanum, then inspect the hypotympanum

This procedure should be done with a 30° scope, with the angle of the endoscope and the posteroinferior part of the specimen facing forward away from the surgeon (**Fig. 19**).

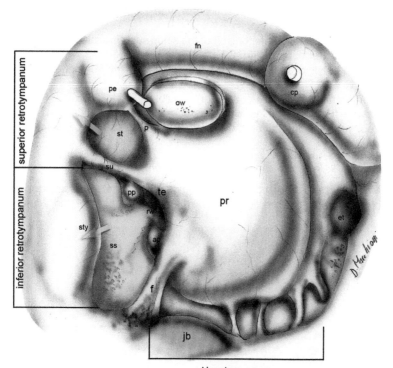

Hypotympanum

Fig. 19. Right ear: Summary of the anatomy of retrotympanum and hypotympanum. Finiculus appears as a ridge of bone arising from the anterior and inferior lip of the round window separating inferior retrotympanum from hypotympanum. Subiculum separates superior from inferior retrotympanum. The *arrows* represents Retrofacial extentions of the sinus tympani and subtympanic sinus. Right side. ap, anterior pillar; cp, cochleariform process; et, eustachian tube; f, finiculus; fn, facial nerve; jb, jugular bulb; ow, oval window; p, ponticulus; pe, pyramidal eminence; pp, posterior pillar; pr, promontory; rw, round window; st, sinus tympani; ss, sinus subtympanicus; su, subiculum; sty, styloid eminence; te, tegmen of round window niche.

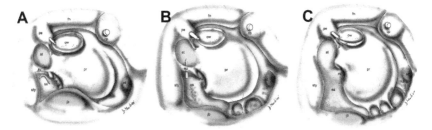

Fig. 20. Right ear: Anatomic variations of the subiculum. (*A*) Ridge subiculum. (*B*) Bridge subiculum. (*C*) Absent subiculum, sinus subtympanicus confluent to the sinus tympani. (*curved arrow*), "dam like" subiculum; (*straight arrow*), "bridge like" subiculum. cp, cochleariform process; et, eustachian tube; fn, facial nerve; jb, jugular bulb; ow, oval window; p, ponticulus; pe, pyramidal eminence; pr, promontory; rw, round window; ss, sinus subtympanicus; st, sinus tympani; su, subiculum; sty, styloid eminence; rw, round window.

Observe

i. Study the anatomy of the subiculum and its different variations (**Fig. 20**).

ii. Observe the subiculum, the inferior limit of the sinus tympani, and the superior limit of the sinus subtympanicus. Identify the type of subiculum in your specimen (**Fig. 21**).

iii. Identify the finiculus, the inferior limit of the sinus subtympanicus. Note the type of finiculus in your specimen (**Fig. 22**).

iv. Observe the styloid eminence, basically delineating the vertical segment of the facial nerve (see **Fig. 21**).

v. Look for the height and size of the jugular bulb.

vi. Take a wide field view and inspect the infracochlear space. If this area is well pneumatized, you can almost see the curvature of the basal turn of the cochlea (see **Fig. 21**).

Dissection Task 9: Initiate a careful limited atticotomy

Make sure that you stop at the insertion point of the lateral incudomallear ligament and the lateral mallear ligament on the medial aspect of the scutum. This

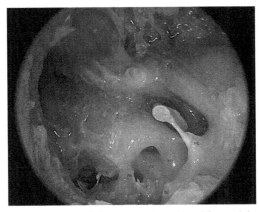

Fig. 21. Left ear: Overview picture of the tympanic cavity with special attention to the retrotympanum. CA, carotid artery; FN, finiculus; FN, facial nerve; HC, hypotympanic air cell; RW, round window; SE, styloid eminence; SS, sinus subtympanicus; SU, subiculum.

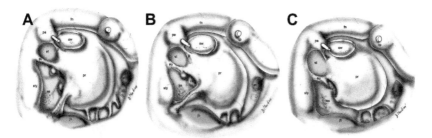

Fig. 22. Anatomic variations of the finiculus. Right side. (*A*) Ridge finiculus. (*B*) Bridge finiculus. (*C*) Absent finiculus. cp, cochleariform process; et, eustachian tube; f, finiculus; fn, facial nerve; jb, jugular bulb; ow, oval window; p, ponticulus; pe, pyramidal eminence; pr, promontory; rw, round window; ss, sinus subtympanicus; st, sinus tympani; su, subiculum; sty, styloid eminence.

procedure needs to be done carefully and in small steps to preserve these friable ligaments.

Observe

i. The shape of the lateral ligaments and how they form, along with the neck of malleus the roof and medial aspect of the Prussak space (**Fig. 23**).
ii. Observe that these ligaments form the lateral part of the epitympanic diaphragm that close up the area in between the scutum and ossicles and prevent any ventilation of the attic via this lateral route. Observe the straight insertion points on the ossicles of the lateral incudomallear ligament and the curvilinear insertion of the lateral mallear ligament (**Fig. 24**).

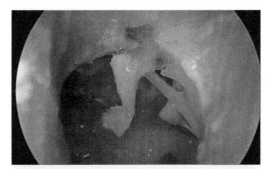

Fig. 23. Left ear: PML, posterior mallear ligament; PR, Prussak space.

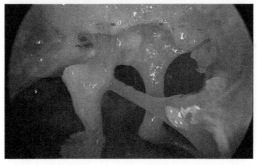

Fig. 24. Left ear: The relatively straight insertion line of the lateral incudomallear ligament (IML) and the downward sloping insertion line of the lateral mallear ligament (LML).

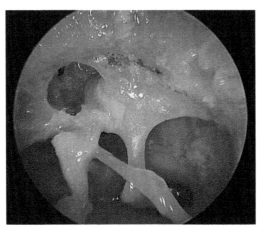

Fig. 25. Left ear: view of the anterior epitympanic space (AES) after removal of the scutum. Note that there is no direct ventilation anteriorly to the eustachian tube.

Dissection Task 10: Continue and extent the atticotomy

Interrupt the lateral mallear fold and curette the anterior part of the scutum and expose the malleus while preserving the incudal part of the lateral incudomallear folds (**Fig. 25**).

Observe

i. Look anterior to the head of malleus for the anterior epitympanic space (see **Fig. 25**). Observe how in most specimens, this space is separated from the supratubal recess by the cog and the tensor folds, which bridge the space between the tensor tympani tendon and the cog.

ii. Look for the presence of Sheehy's cog and complete tensor folds, separating this space from a supratubal recess (**Fig. 26**).

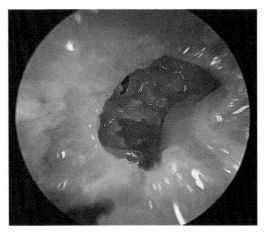

Fig. 26. Left ear: Close-up examination of the anterior epitympanic space (AES). Note that there is no direct ventilation anteriorly to the eustachian tube.

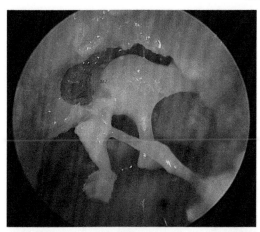

Fig. 27. Left ear: The ossicles are fully exposed within the attic and the incudomallear articulation line is visible. AES, anterior epitympanic space; COG: Sheehy's cog, separating the supratubal recess from the anterior epitympanic space; IMJ, incudomallear joint; TF, tensor folds, partially seen and closing off the attic from direct ventilation into the supratubal recess and the eustachian tube.

Dissection Task 11: Remove entire scutum

Continue on with the removal of the whole scutum along with the lateral incudomallear folds and the exposure of the whole incus and the head of malleus (**Fig. 27**).

Dissection Task 12: Extend the bone removal anteriorly along the anterior bony annulus

Create enough space to introduce your 3-mm angled scope in between the handle of the malleus and bony annulus. Then inspect anteriorly, superiorly, and posteriorly (**Fig. 28**).

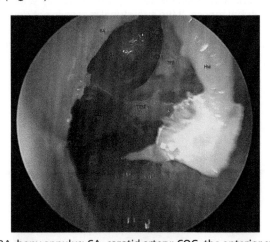

Fig. 28. Left ear: BA, bony annulus; CA, carotid artery; COG, the anterior surface of Sheehy's cog, which separates the attic from the supratubal recess; ET, eustachian tube; HM, handle of malleus; STS, supratubal recess; TFA, the vertical segment of the tensor fold, which when complete, will close off the attic from the eustachian tube; TFB, the horizontal segment of the tensor fold, which forms a partial floor of the supratubal recess anteriorly; TTM, tensor tympani muscle's bony encasement.

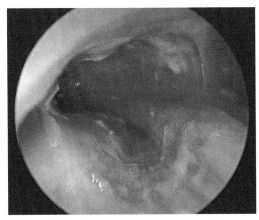

Fig. 29. Left ear: Looking down the eustachian tube. CA, Carotid artery; ET, eustachian tube; STS, supratubal recess; TTM, tensor tympani muscle's bony encasement.

Observe

i. Look down the eustachian tube. Observe the relationship between the carotid artery and the bony encasement of the tensor tympani muscle (**Fig. 29**).

ii. You can use a 45° or 70° scope to look further down the eustachian tube and sometimes be able to identify the actual opening into the nasopharynx (**Fig. 30**).

iii. Rotate your angled scope more superiorly to inspect the size and depth of the supratubal recess, which varies tremendously in size and development. The size of the supratubal recess does not correlate to the degree of pneumatization of the mastoid cavity and attic (**Fig. 31**).

iv. Rotate further superiorly and posteriorly and observe the tensor fold, which when complete separates the anterior attic from the supratubal recess. The shape and position of the tensor fold seems to vary tremendously and are related to the size of the supratubal recess. If the supratubal recess is not developed, the tensor fold is almost a horizontal structure that closes up the anterior attic and separates it from the eustachian tube. It starts with the tendon of the tensor tympani and inserts

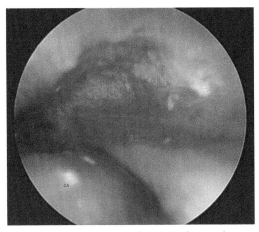

Fig. 30. Using a 45° scope, the opening of the eustachian tube to the nasopharynx is observed. CA, carotid artery; TTM, tensor tympani muscle.

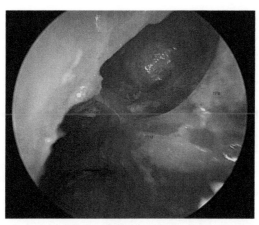

Fig. 31. Left ear: The anatomy of the tensor fold in a specimen with a well-developed supratubal recess. The tensor fold is comprised of 2 segments: a vertical part that attaches to the COG and a horizontal part that forms a partial floor of the supratubal recess. COG, the surface of Sheehy's cog, which separates the supratubal recess from the anterior attic; STS, supratubal recess; TFA, the vertical segment of the tensor fold, which when complete, will close off the attic from the eustachian tube; TFB, the horizontal segment of the tensor fold, which forms a partial floor of the supratubal recess anteriorly; TTM, tensor tympani muscle's bony encasement.

along the ridge of bone formed by the encasement of the tensor tympani muscle and almost into the anterior spine, as in **Figs. 32** and **33**. If the supratubal recess is developed, as in the anatomic specimen featured in this manual, then the tensor fold has 2 parts: the almost vertical part that attaches to the cog and forms with the wall between the supratubal recess and the anterior attic and a horizontal segment that attaches to the tensor tendon and the last part of the ridge formed by the bony encasement of the tensor muscle. In these cases, the horizontal part of the tensor fold forms a partial floor of the supratubal recess (see **Fig. 31**). Alternatively, you can think of the well-developed supratubal recess that has ballooned into the tensor fold and shaped it into these 2 segments (**Fig. 34**).

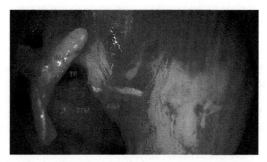

Fig. 32. Right ear: Poorly developed supratubal recess in a surgical case. Using a 70° endoscope and looking up and backward. The tensor fold in these settings is almost a horizontal structure. ABA, anterior bony annulus; HM, handle of malleus; TF, tensor fold; TTM, tensor tympani muscle.

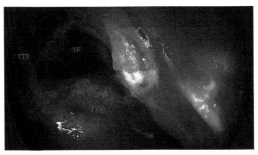

Fig. 33. Right ear: Close-up view of the tensor fold seen in **Fig. 32**. *Red arrow* represents the eustachian tube; TF, tensor fold; TTM, tensor tympani muscle bony encasement; TTT, tensor tympani tendon inserting on the neck of the malleus.

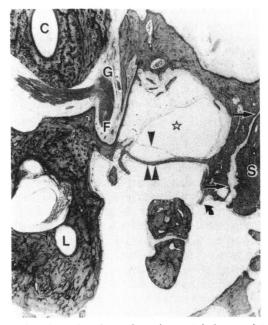

Fig. 34. Histologic section through a dome-shaped supratubal recess (*star*). Straight arrows indicate the outermost plate of the petrosa; curved arrow indicates a spur projecting toward the mallear head to which is attached a mucosal fold associated with the anterior mallear ligament; double arrowheads indicate the cog; and single arrowhead indicates the tensor tympani folds; C, cochlea; F, facial nerve; G, geniculate ganglion; L, lateral semicircular canal; S, scutum.

v. Given that the lateral attic space is closed off by the lateral mallear and incudomallear folds, and a complete tensor fold blocks any direct ventilation through the anterior attic, observe that the only area for epitympanic ventilation is the isthmus, which falls in between the incudostapedial joint and the tensor tendon (**Fig. 35**).

Dissection Task 13: View the articular surface

Push on the incus to view the articular surface with the malleus and with the stapes. Then proceed through with the disarticulation from the stapes and the malleus and the removal of the incus (**Fig. 36**).

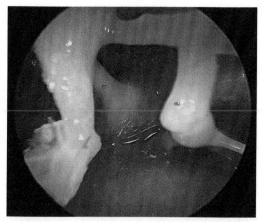

Fig. 35. Left ear: The isthmus forms the only pathway for attic ventilation in the presence of a complete tensor fold. ISJ, incudostapedial joint; TT, tensor tympani tendon.

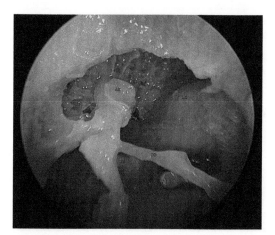

Fig. 36. Left ear: The incus has been removed. AA, aditus antrum; as, articular surface of the head of malleus; CD, chorda tympani; FN, horizontal segment of the facial nerve; SC, lateral semicircular canal; TT, tensor tympani tendon.

Observe

i. The horizontal segment of the facial nerve and the second genu
ii. The lateral semicircular canal
iii. The remnant of the separated attachment of the superior incudal ligament to the attic (**Fig. 37**)

Dissection Task 14: Transect the neck of the malleus

Using a malleus nipper, transect the neck of the malleus at a relatively superior level to preserve the anterior mallear ligament and the tensor tendon to the handle and the neck of the malleus. Remove the head of malleus with the preservation of the ligaments supporting the handle. Pull the handle forward (**Fig. 38**).

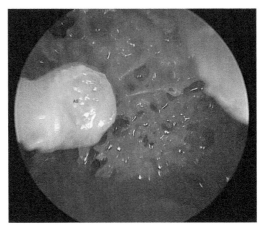

Fig. 37. Left ear: Attic after removal of the incus. As, articular surface of the head of malleus. SL, remnant of the superior ligament of the incus attaching to the tegmen.

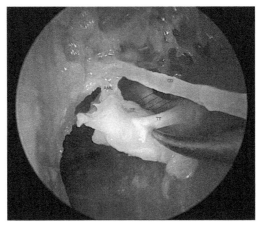

Fig. 38. Left ear: The handle of malleus is pulled forward to demonstrate the tensor fold that had broken of its attachments; the starting points of the arrows indicate the original position of the fold and the ending points indicate the present point after pulling laterally on the handle of malleus. AML, anterior mallear ligament; CD, chorda tympani; TF, tensor fold broken off its original position; TT, tensor tympani tendon.

Observe

  i. The tensor tympani tendon attachment to the neck of the malleus
 ii. The broken of vertical segment of the tensor fold
iii. The course of the chorda tympani
 iv. The anterior reentry of the chorda tympani into its bony canal
  v. The relationship of the chorda to the anterior mallear ligament
 vi. The anterior spine and the attachment of the anterior mallear ligament

Dissection Task 15:

Transect the tensor tympani tendon and remove the handle of malleus (**Fig. 39**).

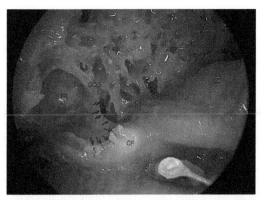

Fig. 39. Left ear: The tensor tendon is transected and the handle of the malleus is removed, so was the anterior spine, anterior mallear ligament, and the chorda tympani. Single arrows indicate the insertion point of the partially removed vertical segment of the tensor fold; double arrows indicate the insertion point of the completely removed horizontal segment of the tensor fold. 1G, first genu of the facial nerve and neighboring geniculate ganglion; CG, cochleariform process; COG, Sheehy's cog; ET, eustachian tube; LC, lateral semicircular canal; STR, supratubal recess; TM, remnant tensor fold.

Observe

i. You can almost see the fibers of the horizontal segment of the facial nerve and the first genu of the nerve as it turns and comes out of the internal Acoustic Meatus (IAC).

ii. Observe the relationship of the cog to the facial nerve's geniculate ganglion.

iii. Observe the remnant of the tensor fold.

iv. Observe the relationship between the second genu of the facial nerve and the lateral semicircular canal (**Fig. 40**).

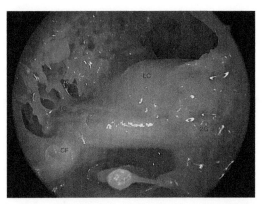

Fig. 40. Left ear: The horizontal segment of the facial nerve and its relationship to the lateral semicircular canal. CH, cochleariform process; LC, lateral canal; 1G, first genu; 2G, second genu.

Elective tasks

> Using a curette or a drill if available, try to slowly remove the bony encasement of the facial nerve starting with the horizontal segment and following the nerve proximally and distally into the first and second genus.

Observe

i. Observe the acute angle of the first genu and the upward kink in that area.
ii. Observe the thin wall of the bone covering the facial nerve especially over the geniculate ganglion, which forms the medial wall of the attic at the area of the cog.
iii. Try to observe the takeoff point from the facial nerve of the first genu of the greater superficial petrosal nerve.
iv. Try to observe the takeoff point of the small nerve supplying the stapedius muscle off the facial nerve after removing its bony encasement through its vertical segment.

17. Using a curette, remove the round window niche. Remove the round window membrane, and enlarge the round window inferiorly and anteriorly to expose the beginning of the scala tympani and the basal turn of the cochlea.

Observe

i. The relationship to the round window to the scala tympani and the slight angulation present
ii. The basal membrane and its pigmentation.

Endoscopic Management of Chronic Otitis Media and Tympanoplasty

Muaaz Tarabichi, MD[a],*, Stéphane Ayache, MD[b],
João Flávio Nogueira, MD[c], Munahi Al Qahtani, MD[d],
David D. Pothier, MBChB, MSc, FRCS(ORL-HNS)[e]

KEYWORDS

- Tympanoplasty • Endoscope • Tympanic perforations • Chronic otitis media

KEY POINTS

- The endoscope allows for better inspection for cholesteatoma in cases with chronic otitis media.
- The endoscope increases the odds of preoperative detection of ossicular chain disruption associated with perforations.
- The endoscope allows better access to selective epitympanic poor ventilation and secondary selective chronic otitis media.
- The endoscope allows for better visualization of anterior poor ventilation of the mesotympanum and reestablishes adequate ventilation to the mesotympanum.
- The endoscope allows better visualization and reconstruction of anterior tympanic membrane perforations.
- The endoscope allows use of Sheehy's lateral graft tympanoplasty through a transcanal approach.

Videos of endoscopic detection of stapedial reflexes; endoscopic medial graft tympanoplasty with ossicular reconstruction; two for endoscopic medial graft tympanoplasty; endoscopic butterfly button tympanoplasty; endoscopic lateral graft tympanoplasty; and interlay tympanoplasty techniques accompany this article at http://www.oto.theclinics.com/

Disclosures: No disclosures.
[a] Center for Ear Endoscopy, Kenosha, WI, USA; [b] Department of Otolaryngology, ORPAC, Clinique du Palais, Grasse, France; [c] Department of Otolaryngology, Hospital Geral de Fortaleza, Fortaleza, Brazil; [d] Department of Otolaryngology, Riyadh Military Hospital, Riyadh, Saudi Arabia; [e] Department of Otolaryngology Head and Neck Surgery, Toronto General Hospital, University Health Network and University of Toronto, Ontario, Canada
* Corresponding author.
E-mail address: tarabichi@yahoo.com

INTRODUCTION

As discussed in the article elsewhere in this issue by Tarabachi, Marchioni, Presutti, and Nogueira, Endoscopic Transcanal Ear Anatomy and Dissection, the endoscope allows greater access to the tympanic cavity[1] and therefore offers a fresh outlook on conditions that affect this space and offers distinct advantages in the understanding of this condition and the management of its sequela.

ASSESSING STATUS OF MIDDLE EAR VENTILATION

Although the cause of chronic otitis media without chlolesteatoma is poorly understood, poor ventilation of the different air spaces within the temporal bone is believed to be at the center of this disease process. Combined tympanomastoidectomy with exenteration of air cells is considered the treatment of choice. Failure to exenterate tegmental cells from disease is a common cause of failure.[2] The endoscope allows for expanded access to the attic, especially anteriorly, and this allows for removal of any granulation tissue in that area.[1] Beyond any Eustachian tube dysfunction, there are multiple opportunities for obstruction within the narrow ventilation pathways of the tympanic cavity, which result in selective poor ventilation of the areas proximal to these sites. The 2 main areas lie anteriorly within the anterior mesotympanum and posteriorly and superiorly within the epitympanic diaphragm, 2 areas that are more accessible with the endoscope.[1] Classic surgical approaches to the attic with microscopic transmastoid technique results in poor access to the anterior attic and extensive removal of much of the associated anatomy to access these areas. In contrast, the endoscope offers clear glimpses of the anatomy and disease without undue disruption of the anatomy, making it easier to understand both the underlying anatomy and any disease process within this area.[1–6] This situation is particularly true when considering the tensor fold. Because of the location and orientation of this fold, it is a structure that cannot be seen through traditional microscopic transcanal and transmastoid approaches to the anterior attic.[7] The only exception to this situation is a widely opened facial recess, and only after removal of the incus. It is often helpful to push the handle of malleus laterally for a more open view. This observation of the tensor fold is usually made more difficult while operating on diseased ears because of the existing medialization of the handle of malleus and the fact that blood tends to pool in this area because of the position of the head in traditional mastoid surgery. The endoscope allows for inspection of this fold in healthy ears by using a 30° endoscope and looking through the isthmus (**Fig. 1**). In diseased ears, the isthmus is obstructed and narrow because of medialization of the handle of malleus, and the tensor fold can be visualized endoscopically either by looking superiorly and posteriorly with an angled scope that is positioned anterior to the handle of malleus (**Fig. 2**) or by looking forward with an angled scope after removal of the incus and ahead of malleus (**Fig. 3**).

Examination of the tympanic cavity in the clinic through perforations is helpful in assessing the status of the middle ear mucosa beyond the perforation and the presence of inflammatory webs in the anterior epitympanum as well as any obstruction of the isthmus, which can result in recurrent episodes of drainage or poor response to local treatment.[3] The endoscope allows for better surgical access to the tensor fold and the anterior epitympanic space to establish ventilation without disrupting the ossicular chain.[1]

ASSESSING THE STATUS OF THE OSSICULAR CHAIN

The incudostapedial joint and the stapes suprastructure are almost universally accessible for inspection endoscopically through a perforation or a thin retracted

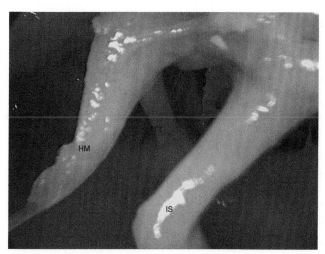

Fig. 1. Right ear: peaking through the isthmus with a 30° endoscope. CO, COG; HM, handle of malleus; IS, incudostapedial joint; RE, the recess formed through the insertion of the fold anterior to the COG; TF, tensor fold; TT, tendon of the tensor tympani.

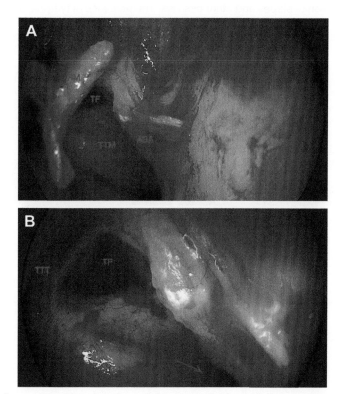

Fig. 2. Right ear intraoperative view of the tensor fold, which has an almost-horizontal orientation without any formation of supratubal recess. (*A*) General view; (*B*) close-up view. ABA, anterior bony annulus; *arrow*, Eustachian tube; HM, handle of malleus; TF, horizontal tensor fold; TTM, tensor tympani muscle canal; TTT, tendon of the tensor tympani.

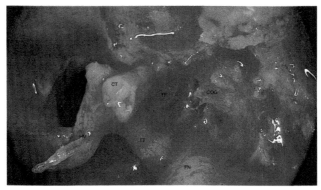

Fig. 3. Left ear intraoperative view. The incus and the head of malleus is removed and looking forward with a 30° scope toward the anterior attic at a tensor fold with almost-vertical orientation. COG, COG; CT, transected corda tympani; FN, horizontal segment of the facial nerve; HM, handle of malleus; TF, tensor fold; TT, tensor tympani tendon.

membrane.[8] Even with the use of a 0° endoscope, the endoscopic view allows for a better inspection of the ossicles (**Fig. 4**). The lack of stapedial reflexes in the presence of an intact tympanic membrane and good bone thresholds had been a useful way of detecting fixation of stapes and other ossicles. The presence of tymphanic membrane

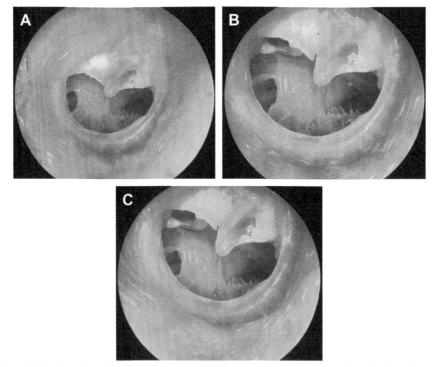

Fig. 4. (A) Overall endoscopic picture of perforation that is without the visualization of ossicular chain, probably similar to what is visible with microscope. (B) Close-up endoscopic view with visualization of the stapes. (C) Further close-up view showing the incudostapedial joint; all with 0° endoscopes.

perforation precludes this useful test. Endoscopic detection of stapedial reflexes through perforations allows for the identification of stapes fixation.[9] It also tests the integrity of an eroded, visually connected incudostapedial joint (Video 1).

ENDOSCOPIC MEDIAL GRAFT TYMPANOPLASTY

Medial graft tympanoplasty is a common and relatively successful procedure; central to its success is adequate and relatively free exposure to the whole tympanic perforation. Unfavorable ear canal anatomy (overhanging anterior wall or a small canal) or anterior perforations make for a technically challenging transcanal procedure, which is reflected as a high rate of failure. Experience surgeons are usually more willing to consider a postauricular approach in these limiting situations to provide adequate microscopic exposure.[10]

OPERATIVE TECHNIQUE FOR ENDOSCOPIC MEDIAL GRAFT TYMPANOPLASTY

- The ear canal and the graft donor site are infiltrated with xylocaine 2% with 1 in 100,000 epinephrine (Videos 2, 3 and 4).
- A fascial graft is obtained from either the temporalis muscle fascia or tragal perichondrium.
- The edges of the perforation are debrided and the undersurface of the tympanic membrane is abraded.
- A wide tympanomeatal flap is elevated.
- The ossicular chain is inspected either through the perforation or directly after elevation of the tympanomeatal flap.
- Appropriate ossicular reconstruction is performed.
- The graft is positioned just medial to the anterior rim of the perforation as it is visualized through the tympanomeatal flap.
- If the anterior rim is not visible through the elevated flap, then a 30° endoscope is used to perform that step and to pack Gelfoam (Pfizer Canada Inc., Quebec, Canada) in the middle ear deep to the graft.
- The tympanomeatal flap is repositioned and the ear canal is packed with Gelfoam.

The impact of the endoscope on tympanoplasty surgery needs to be considered based on the surgical task contemplated and the importance of the advantages and disadvantages in specific situations, such as:

1. Elevation of tympanomeatal flap: this is performed under direct vision with the endoscope without the need for the continuous repositioning in microscopic surgery. It is difficult to tear a flap because the angle of view includes both surfaces of the whole flap. It is easy to identify and cauterize bleeding points along the incised edge of the skin of the ear canal.
2. Inspection of the middle ear space: the endoscope is the better instrument here for the reasons discussed earlier. This inspection includes operative evaluation and treatment of disease within the facial recess, sinus tympani, hypotympanum, attic, and the anterior part of the tympanic cavity.
3. Positioning of the graft: this task is easier with the endoscope, given its wide angle of view, which includes the tympanic ring along with the whole perforation and graft without the need for repositioning.
4. Positioning of a prosthesis: the unavailability of 2 hands (eg, to lift malleus) and the lack of depth perception (assessing length of prosthesis needed) makes this task more difficult with the endoscope.

5. Butterfly button tympanoplasty with an anterior perforation is a particularly manageable technique with the endoscope (Video 5).

It is difficult to use the endoscope and microscope to perform different tasks in the same procedure, and different surgeons choose their instrument of choice based on their comfort level.

The first report of endoscopic medial graft tympanoplasty in 1998 showed a high success rate in 64 ears.[11] The main point to be emphasized is how endoscopic techniques reduced the rate of postauricular approach from 42% (before the use of the endoscope) to 0%, without reducing the overall success rate and without increasing the complication rate. The first author of this article has not performed any postauricular or endaural incisions for tympanic perforations since that report.

Despite the safety of endoscopic ossicular chain reconstruction, there are no compelling reasons for performing ossicular work with the endoscope.

ENDOSCOPIC LATERAL GRAFT TYMPANOPLASTY

A wide and complete view of the tympanic ring is an essential element in Sheehy's lateral graft tympanoplasty.[12] This view is usually accomplished by enlarging the ear canal and through postauricular exposure. The endoscope offers a comparable wide view of the operative field through a transcanal approach.

OPERATIVE TECHNIQUE FOR ENDOSCOPIC LATERAL GRAFT TYMPANOPLASTY

- The ear canal and the graft donor site are infiltrated with xylocaine 2% with 1 in 100,000 epinephrine (Video 6).
- A fascial graft is obtained from either the temporalis muscle fascia or tragal perichondrium.
- The skin of the ear canal is removed along with the epithelial layer of the tympanic membrane remnant. The vascular strip is preserved.
- Overhanging bony ear canal is curetted out to obtain full endoscopic exposure to the anterior sulcus.
- The ossicular chain is inspected either through the perforation or directly after elevation of annulus if there is strong suspicion of disease based on preoperative audiogram.
- Appropriate ossicular reconstruction is performed, the middle ear cavity is packed with Gelfoam, and the facial graft and the skin are repositioned. The ear canal is packed with Gelfoam.

The usefulness of the endoscope in lateral graft tympanoplasty must be considered based on the surgical task contemplated and the importance of the advantages and disadvantages in specific situations:

1. Removal of canal skin: the use of the endoscope allows canal skin to be removed under direct vision without the usual need for continuous manipulation of the microscope. It is difficult to tear the skin because the angle of view includes both surfaces. It is easy to identify and cauterize bleeding points at the edges of the incised skin as well as any anterior sulcus perforator vessels, which usually produce significant bleeding.
2. Drilling and removal of overhanging bony canal: the ability to visualize past the shaft of the drill into the surgical field makes the endoscope a useful instrument. The wide angle of view of the endoscope might lead the surgeon to underestimate the depth

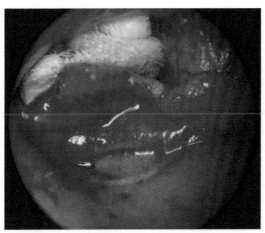

Fig. 5. Interlay tympanoplasty of left ear: the squamous layer is elevated off the fibrous layer of the tympanic membrane, leaving the fibrous layer in situ.

of the anterior sulcus, which could lead to inadequate removal of overhanging bony canal, which results in blunting of the anterior sulcus.
3. Inspection of the middle ear space: the endoscope is the better instrument here for the enhanced visualization described earlier.
4. Positioning of the graft: this task is easier with the endoscope, given its wide angle of view, which includes the whole tympanic ring.

The first report of endoscopic lateral graft tympanoplasty in 1998 showed a high success rate in 32 ears, with 3 patients having blunting of the anterior sulcus and 1 patient having a cholesteatoma pearl within the tympanic membrane at 1 year post-operatively.[11] The primary investigator of that study has since relied more on this technique to improve success rate in tympanoplasty surgery.

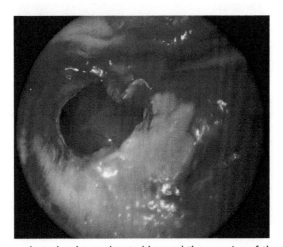

Fig. 6. The squamous layer has been elevated beyond the margins of the perforation.

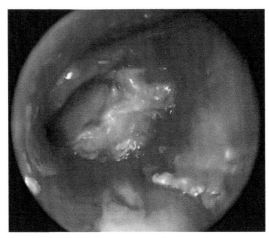

Fig. 7. A graft is inserted between the squamous layer and the fibrous layer and the flap replaced.

INTERLAY TYMPANOPLASTY

Most perforations of the tympanic membrane that are not associated with ossicular abnormalities or the ingress of keratin into the middle ear are closed with an underlay graft or a lateral graft tympanoplasty. The former is easier to perform, but the graft lacks the support of the fibrous layer of the tympanic membrane remnant; the latter provides a more robust support for the graft, but comes at the price of a substantial amount of trauma to the skin of the ear canal that is explanted and replaced as part of this procedure. This situation can cause blunting of the anterior recess of the external ear canal and may cause problems with the transfer of sound energy.

Using an endoscopic approach, it is possible to perform a hybrid technique that has not been easy to perform with the microscope, because of the difficulty with access to

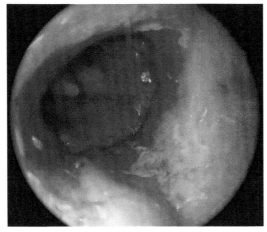

Fig. 8. The graft is now sandwiched between the fibrous and the squamous layer, which provides a robust support for the graft.

the anterior region of the tympanic membrane. The hybrid interlay technique involves the raising of an extended tympanomeatal flap to the level of the fibrous annulus of the tympanic membrane. At this point, rather than raising the flap along with the annulus and the tympanic membrane, the squamous layer is elevated off the fibrous layer of the tympanic membrane, leaving the fibrous layer in situ (**Fig. 5**). After the squamous layer has been elevated beyond the margins of the perforation (**Fig. 6**), a graft is inserted between the squamous layer and the fibrous layer and the flap replaced (**Fig. 7**). The graft material can be temporalis fascia, perichondrium, or a composite graft.

The graft is now sandwiched between the fibrous and the squamous layer, which provides a robust support for the graft (**Fig. 8**). This technique preserves the integrity of the fibrous annulus and leaves the skin of the ear canal in position in the anterior recess and still provides a stable bed for the graft. A potential drawback is the difficulty in raising the squamous layer from the fibrous layer, but this is easier to perform with wide access to the flap and the accurate and highly magnified view of the interface of these layers afforded by the endoscopic view (Video 7).

SUPPLEMENTARY DATA

Supplementary data related to this article can be found online at http://dx.doi.org/10.1016/j.otc.2012.12.002.

REFERENCES

1. Tarabichi M. Transcanal endoscopic management of cholesteatoma. Otol Neurotol 2010;31:580–8.
2. Nadol JB. Causes of failure of mastoidectomy for chronic otitis media. Laryngoscope 1985;95:410–3.
3. Mansour S, Nicolas K, Naim A, et al. Inflammatory chronic otitis media and the anterior epitympanic recess. J Otolaryngol 2005;34(3):149–59.
4. Tarabichi M. Endoscopic management of acquired cholesteatoma. Am J Otol 1997;18:544–9.
5. Tarabichi M. Endoscopic management of cholesteatoma: long-term results. Otolaryngol Head Neck Surg 2000;122:874–81.
6. Tarabichi M. Endoscopic management of limited attic cholesteatoma. Laryngoscope 2004;114:1157–62.
7. Marchioni D, Alicandri-Ciufelli M, Molteni M. Selective dysventilation syndrome. Laryngoscope 2010;120:1028–33.
8. Karhuketo TS, Puhakka HJ, Laippala PJ. Tympanoscopy to increase the accuracy of diagnosis in conductive hearing loss. J Laryngol Otol 1998;112(2):154–7.
9. Al-Qahtani MM, Hagr AA. A preliminary study of endoscopic acoustic stapedial reflex in chronic otitis media. Saudi Med J 2010;31(8):900–3.
10. Doyle PJ, Schleuning AJ, Echevarria J. Tympanoplasty: should grafts be placed medial or lateral to the tympanic membrane? Laryngoscope 1972;82:1425–30.
11. Tarabichi M. Endoscopic middle ear surgery. Ann Otol Rhinol Laryngol 1999;108:39–46.
12. Sheehy JL. Surgery of chronic otitis media. In: English GM, editor. Otolaryngology. New York: Harper and Row; 1977.

Endoscopic Anatomy and Ventilation of the Epitympanum

Daniele Marchioni, MD*, Alessia Piccinini, MD,
Matteo Alicandri-Ciufelli, MD, Livio Presutti, MD

KEYWORDS

- Endoscopic ear surgery • Epitympanum • Middle ear ventilation • Surgical anatomy
- Prussak space

KEY POINTS

- The superior attic (upper unit) is in communication with the mesotympanum through the underlying tympanic isthmus and posteriorly it is open to the aditus ad antrum.
- The inferior lateral attic and the Prussack space are lower than the epitympanic diaphragm, and it is ventilated by the mesotympanum.
- An isthmus blockage associated with a complete tensor fold leads to inadequate ventilation of the mastoid cells and this scenario could be at the basis of the attic retraction pocket development.
- During surgery, in sectorial disventilatory disorders caused by isthmus block, it is essential to restore the ventilation pathway through the isthmus and to create an alternative direct ventilatory route between the protympanum and anterior attic from a section of the central portion of the tensor fold.
- Endoscopic middle ear surgery may help in understanding the physiopathology of the middle ear, allowing the surgeon to explore middle ear anatomy, and thus all ventilation pathways.

INTRODUCTION

Aeration of the tympanic cavity and mastoid cells and anatomic pathways for middle ear ventilation have been studied since the end of the nineteenth century, starting with the work of Prussak[1] in 1867. More recently, Palva and Johnsson[2] were the first to describe middle ear anatomy focusing on ventilation patterns and their implications for middle ear disease.

The eustachian tube (ET) plays a crucial role in maintaining middle ear aeration and atmospheric pressure. Inflammatory middle ear chronic disease is usually related to

---

Disclosures: All of the authors have read and approved the manuscript. None of the authors have any financial relationships to disclose.
Conflict of interest: None.
Otolaryngology, Head and Neck Surgery Department, Policlinic of Modena, University Hospital of Modena, Via del Pozzo 71, Modena 41100, Italy
* Corresponding author.
E-mail address: marchionidaniele@yahoo.it

ET dysfunction caused by poor tympanic ventilation. This condition is also related to hearing impairment and poor postoperative outcomes.[3] Although middle ear aeration is related to ET function, other anatomic factors may play important roles in ventilation of these spaces and, in particular, in the pathophysiology of selective epitympanic retraction.

In recent years, the use of endoscope with varied angulations has allowed the surgeon to explore all of the hidden areas that are often not visualized using a micro-scope.[4–7] Endoscopes have also improved knowledge of the complex fold anatomy and functional interventions in middle ear inflammatory disorders during middle ear surgery, particularly in the case of selective dysventilation.[8]

This article discusses the anatomy of the epitympanum and the ventilation patterns and pathophysiology of epitympanic retraction.

The Epitympanic Compartments (Anterior and Posterior Epitympanum) and the Concept of Upper and Lower Units

The epitympanum is divided into 2 compartments: a large posterior compartment and a smaller anterior compartment. The demarcation between the anterior and posterior epitympanum depends on the anatomic variations of important structures such as the cog and the tensor fold. In most people, the demarcation between the anterior and posterior epitympanum is represented by the transverse ridge or cog. The cog is a bony septum that detaches from the tegmen tympani cranially, leading vertically toward the cochleariform process in front of the malleus head.

Much of the posterior epitympanic volume is occupied by the body and short process of the incus together with the head of the malleus. The lateral portion of the posterior epitympanum is narrow and is divided by the lateral incudomalleolar fold in 2 further portions, the superior and inferior lateral attic, positioned separately one above the other.

The incudomalleolar fold originates at the posterior extremity of the short process of incus and the lateral portion of the posterior incudal fold, continuing anteriorly between the body of the incus, the head of the malleus and the lateral aspect of the attic. At this level, the fold bends inferiorly, joining the posterior malleolar ligament fold and the lateral malleolar ligament fold, with which it forms the medial and superior aspect of the Prussak space (**Fig. 1**).

The inferior lateral attic is bounded superiorly by the lateral incudo-malleolar fold. This anatomic area is therefore in a lower position than the epitympanic diaphragm in communication with the underlying mesotympanum. Ventilation of the inferior lateral attic is provided by the mesotympanic region. In a more cranial position than the inferior lateral attic lies the superior lateral attic, whose floor or inferior limit is represented by the incudomalleolar fold. Together with the medial attic, this anatomic area is called the superior attic or upper unit.

The superior attic is in communication with the mesotympanum through the underlying tympanic isthmus, and posteriorly it is opened to the aditus ad antrum. Its upper limit is the tegmen tympani, the lower limit is the second (intratympanic) portion of the facial nerve, and laterally it is bounded by the bony lateral wall of the atticus. The superior attic is therefore ventilated through the isthmus (**Fig. 2**).

The lower unit is formed by the reduced space represented by the Prussak space, which is separated in its anatomy and ventilation from the upper unit by its vault, represented by the lateral malleolar ligament fold. This inferior epitympanic portion is ventilated in most cases from the posterior pocket through mesotympanum (see **Fig. 1** panel D).

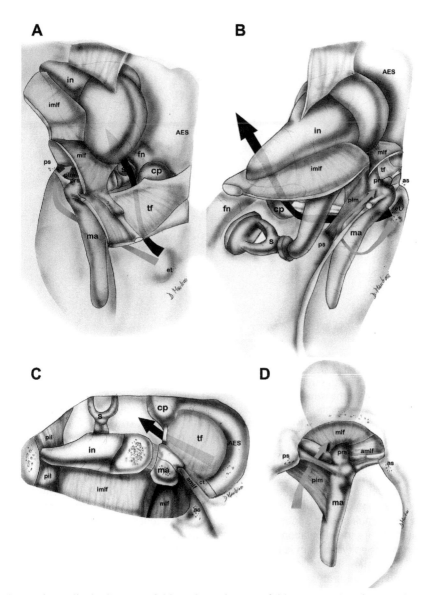

Fig. 1. The malleolar ligament folds and membranous folds representing the complete epitympanic diaphragm, and the 2 major middle ear ventilation pathways of the epitympanic compartments (*blue arrow*) and Prussak space (*orange arrow*). (*A*) Anterior view. (*B*) Posterior view. (*C*) Axial view according to Palva. (*D*) Lateral view of Prussak space. AES, anterior epitympanic space; amlf, anterior malleal ligamental fold; as, anterior spine; bin, body of the incus; cp, cochleariform process; ct, corda tympani; et, eustachian tube; fn, facial nerve; hma, head of the malleus; imlf, lateral incudomalleal fold; in, incus; ma, malleus; mlf, lateral malleal ligamental fold; PES, posterior epitympanic space; pil, lateral and medial posterior incudal ligaments; plm, posterior malleal ligamental fold; prs, Prussak space; ps, posterior spine; s, stapes; sr, supratubal recess; tf, tensor fold. The orange arrow indicates the major ventilation pathway through the posterior pocket.

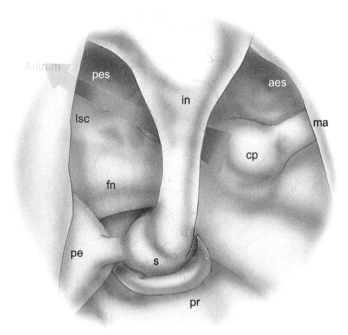

Fig. 2. Right ear. The posterior isthmus after posterior atticotomy maintaining the integrity of the ossicular chain (the red arrow represents the main ventilation route from the ET to the antrum through the isthmus). aes, anterior epitympanic compartment; cp, cochleariform process; fn, facial nerve; in, incus; lsc, lateral semicircular canal; ma, malleus; pe, pyramidal eminence; pes, posterior epitympanic compartment; s, stapes; tf, tensor fold; ttc, tensor tympani canal.

The 2 ventilatory trajectories of the epitympanic units are therefore separated from each other; this pathophysiologic concept is important in transcanalar endoscopic surgery, because surgical treatment is based on the restoration of ventilation and on the unification of the upper unit with the lower unit, through the creation of a large tympanic isthmus and an accessory route through the tensor fold. The surgical solution must ensure the ventilation of all parts of the epitympanum.

The anterior epitympanum is delimited anteriorly by the root of the zygomatic arch (a thick bony plate that separates it from pericarotic cells), superiorly by the tegmen tympani (which separates it from the meninges), laterally by the tympanic bone and chorda tympani, and medially by a bony wall that separates it from the geniculate fossa, which contains the homonymous ganglion. Its inferior limit is represented by the tensor fold, which, if complete, separates it from the underlying sovratubaric recess. The tensor fold presents a variable anatomy: according to Palva and colleagues,[9] the tensor fold is incomplete in only 25% of cases, allowing an alternative ventilation route directed from the sovratubaric recess toward the attic (**Fig. 7**). It extends laterally from the semicanal of the tensor tympani muscle to the lateral aspect of the protympanum, posteriorly adhering to the cochleariform process and to the tensor tympani tendon, and extends anteriorly to the root of the zygomatic bone to provide the epitympanic floor.

If it inserts on the transverse crest, its direction is almost vertical, whereas, if inserts on the tubaric tegmen, its direction is horizontal.

In most cases the curvature is about 45° and its most frequent insertion lies at the central portion of the anterior sovratubaric-epitympanic tegmen. According to our observations on patients affected by attic cholesteatomas, a complete tensor fold has been observed in almost all the patients studied, and the direction of the fold was in most cases horizontal.[4] In general, the width of the underlying sovratubaric recess varies depending on its angle (**Fig. 3**).

During surgery, in sectorial ventilatory disorders caused by isthmus block, it is essential to create an alternative direct ventilatory route between the protympanum and anterior attic from a section of the central portion of the tensor fold.

The anterior epitympanum can be formed from a single large air cell, or by several small air cells, and this makes the anterior epitympanum a variable anatomic space in an anterior-posterior direction. In a recent study conducted at our clinic, subjects affected by cholesteatoma limited to the attic showed a reduced volume of the bony boundaries of the anterior epitympanum. The small anterior epitympanic cavities might be proof of selective attic dysventilation.

Epitympanic Diaphragm and Epitympanic Ventilation Patterns

The concept of epitympanic diaphragm was raised for the first time by Lemoine in 1950;[5] the investigators described that the diaphragm was made up of various structures and membranous ligaments that, together with the malleus and the incus, form the floor of the epitympanic compartment.

The investigators also described the Prussak area as a structure located inferiorly to this diaphragm, therefore dividing it from the epitympanic compartments by the lateral malleolar ligament fold, considered the Prussak space roof.

In addition to the folds described by Lemoine, Palva[2] added 2 more duplicated folds: the tensor fold and the lateral incudomalleolar fold. The complete diaphragm therefore comprises the 3 malleolar ligament folds (anterior, lateral, and posterior),

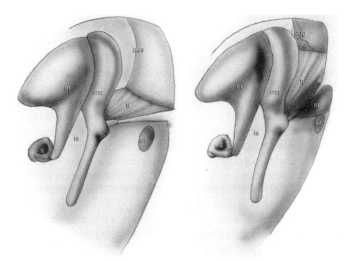

Fig. 3. Right ear. The variations in size of the supratubal recess. The dimensions of this recess depend on the inclination of the tensor fold (*right*). The more vertical the tensor fold, the wider the supratubal recess. When the tensor fold is a horizontal, the supratubal recess is not present (*left*). et, eustachian tube; in, incus; is, isthmus; ma, malleus; s, stapes; sr, supratubal recess; tf, tensor fold.

the posterior incudal fold, and the 2 duplicated membranous folds (tensor fold and the lateral incudomalleolar fold) associated with the incus and the malleus.

Palva classified Proctor's anterior tympanic isthmus as a single entity that is always present, and defined it simply as the tympanic isthmus, whereas the ventilation route posterior to the incus, an irregular feature named by Proctor[6] the posterior isthmus, provides inconsistent ventilation from the fossa incudis.

The tympanic isthmus described by Palva represents a wide ventilation route for the epitympanum, excluding the Prussak space.

This structure extends anteriorly from the tensor fold to the pyramidal process (inferiorly and posteriorly) and to the medial portion of the posterior incus ligament (superiorly and posteriorly). Its medial limit is the attic bony wall and the lateral limit is the body of the incus, the incus short process, and the head of the malleus.

The space bounded by these structures is called the middle attic, which becomes the mesotympanum inferior to the body incus.

The anterior portion of the tympanic isthmus, superior to the level of the tensor tympani tendon, represents a wide communication with the anterior epitympanum. In healthy ears, the tympanic isthmus is an open structure with no fold.

Although Palva noticed a wide opening just behind the incus short process in 25% of Proctor posterior tympanic isthmus, in most cases this potential posterior ventilation route was blocked by the posterior incus ligament fold.

Given this, all the compartments leading to the epitympanic diaphragm receive air through the only ventilation way that is always present, the tympanic isthmus route, located between the medial aspect of the posterior incus ligament and the tensor fold.

However, Palva[2,9] noticed that membranous folds that formed the epitympanic diaphragm could have structural defects resulting in incomplete folds.

In this way, additional ventilation patterns arise for the structures above the epitympanic diaphragm. Most of the defects were of the tensor fold (29% of cases), followed by the lateral incudomalleolar fold in its anterior portion (15% of cases).

The Prussak Space

The medial and inferior aspects of the Prussak space are formed respectively by the neck and the short process of the malleus.

The superior limit is the fold of the lateral malleolar ligament, which also represents the floor of the lateral malleolar space; this ligament inserts laterally on the medial wall of the scutum. The lateral malleolar ligament fold is integral in most case, because according to Palva[9] only 19% of subjects showed a defect in the anterior portion of the fold, whereas, in some rare cases (7% of the subjects examined by Palva), the defect was in the posterior portion of the ligament, the latter involving the lateral malleolar ligament fold, creating a communication between the upper epitympanic portion (upper unit) and the lower (lower unit), resulting in a communication between the Prussak space and the lateral malleolar space and creating a change in the classic epitympanic diaphragm.

The anterior aspect of the Prussak area is bounded by a thin, membranous fold among the tympanic membrane and the anterior malleolar ligament fold, which inserts laterally on the tympanic membrane and medially on the neck and long process of the malleus.

In some cases, this fold is absent, causing a further anterior ventilation trajectory to the Prussak space.

The lateral aspect is represented by the Sharpnell membrane.

The posterior wall is represented by a large posterior pocket (the posterior pocket of von Tröltsch), which is the main route of ventilation. This posterior pocket is bounded laterally by the pars tensa and pars flaccida of the tympanic membrane, and medially by the posterior malleolar ligament fold, which originates from the posterior portion of the malleus neck and the upper third of the malleus handle and inserts posteriorly in the posterior tympanic spine (**Fig. 1**; Panel D). This posterior pocket develops in a posterior-inferior direction and opens at the most cranial portion of mesotympanum, so, in most people, ventilation of the Prussak space occurs through the communication with the mesotympanum, the only ventilation route that is separated from the epitympanic upper unit. This ventilation route of the inferior epitympanic compartment through the posterior pocket of von Tröltsch is rough and narrow, especially compared with the ventilation route through tympanic isthmus, which aerates the upper epitympanic compartment and is wider. For these reasons, the possibility of anatomic reduction of the passage until the closing of the posterior pocket is plausible, especially the presence of thick and viscous secretions within the Prussak space that could cause a chronic sectorial dysventilation associated with a retraction of the Sharpnell membrane and its adhesion with the malleus neck.

For these reasons, although the Prussak space is anatomically inseparable from the epitympanum, in terms of ventilation and drainage, it represents an independent unit.

This space may have a block and/or an obliteration without any involvement of the compartments above the epitympanic diaphragm, like the anterior and posterior epitympanum, the aditus, and mastoid cells.

Palva dissected subjects on ventilation tubes for epitympanic retraction, showed that, despite the surgical treatment, an attical dysventilation was still present.[2]

Given these phenomena, Palva assumed that behind the genesis of attical cholesteatoma there was a progressive closure of the ventilation route of the inferior epitympanic unit (lower unit) initially derived from mucous tissue inflammation in the posterior pocket and Prussack space, then from the granulation tissue formation that progressively causes a total block to the passage of air from this route. These events could lead to retraction of the Sharpnell membrane toward the malleus neck. The positioning of a ventilation tube causes an improvement in mesotympanic and hypotympanic ventilation, but does not address the blockage in the posterior pocket, and the process of retraction would be irreversible. It is still debated whether these phenomena are sufficient to cause an attical cholesteatoma.[10]

DISCUSSION OF MIDDLE EAR ANATOMY

Intraoperative evaluation of middle ear anatomy during endoscopic surgery for inflammatory disorders allows the visualization of anatomic blockages of the middle ear ventilation patterns.

Many other investigators have described the anatomy and development of tympanic compartments and folds because this knowledge is crucial in the understanding and treatment of middle ear disease.

More recently, tympanic isthmus and middle ear ventilation patterns have been described in several articles.

Palva and Johnsson[2,9] studied the anatomy of the tensor fold during temporal bone dissection. They observed that, in most patients, the tensor fold was a complete fold separating the epitympanic compartment from the protympanum. In these patients, the isthmus was the only aeration pathway; however, in rare cases, it is possible to observe an incomplete tensor fold; in these cases, the anterior epitympanic space received aeration directly from the protympanum through the communication in the tensor fold area.

Although exploration of the tensor fold region during middle ear surgery for chronic disease has already been established in the international literature, it is not easy to reach this region in otomicroscopy.

Several approaches have been described in the international literature, but we suggest an endoscopic approach to the tensor fold in patients with attic disease, which could be exclusive or combined with the traditional microscopic approach.[11]

In our previous study[12] focused on epitympanic size in patients affected by a limited attic cholesteatoma, we observed that the anterior epitympanic recess (AER) in an affected ear is smaller than in an unaffected ear. We hypothesized that the presence of a tympanic isthmus blockage associated with a complete tensor fold could exclude the AER from the posterior epitympanic space and from the protympanum. The blockage of the tympanic isthmus could create a selective negative pressure in the atticomastoid spaces; this chronic lack of aeration could provoke a hypodevelopment of the AER with a reduction of pressure level and, consequently, an attic retraction and cholesteatoma sac development (**Fig. 4**). This process is also possible in patients with a normally functioning ET.

Middle Ear Blockage

An isthmus blockage caused by chronic inflammatory disease in association with a complete tensor fold leads to inadequate ventilation of the mastoid cells and epitympanic recess. Middle ear pressure seems related not only to a functioning ET but also to transmucosal gas exchange through the mastoid mucosa. The mucosal gas exchange is related to the degree of mastoid pneumatization.[13] Because of these 2 gas pressure regulation systems, even if the ET is functioning, an isthmus blockage could impair ventilation of the mastoid cells, causing sclerotization of the mastoid. It is not clear whether chronic middle ear disease leads to inadequate mastoid pneumatization or, conversely, a sclerotic mastoid leads to chronic middle ear disease.[14]

In a recent study,[4] we described the kinds of anatomic blockage of the middle ear ventilation trajectories that may be identified during endoscopic surgery to understand whether those alterations could be associated with anomalous mastoid pneumatization, a classic sign of middle ear dysventilation problems.

In this study, the anatomic structure that separates epitympanic space from the mesotympanum (tympanic isthmus and tensor fold area) was studied. No previous studies have been performed on the surgical approach for patients affected by a middle ear chronic disease with blockage of the isthmus. Intraoperative evaluation of middle ear anatomy during endoscopic surgery allowed us to clearly visualize the presence of anatomic blockage of the middle ear ventilation trajectories. We classified these anatomic blockage patterns into 3 types (**Fig. 5**):

- Type A: blockage of the isthmus associated with a complete tensor fold (most of these patients presented a selective attic retraction pocket or attic cholesteatoma without pathologic tissue in the mesotympanic spaces)
- Type B: blockage of the isthmus associated with an attical vertical blockage (consisting of a fold or granulation tissue involving the incudomalleal fold) separating the anterior epitympanic space from the posterior epitympanic space with or without a complete tensor fold, in these subjects a selective retraction pocket into the posterior attic was found
- Type C: a complete epidermization of the attic space causing a blockage of the isthmus and a complete antral blockage excluding the mesotympanic space from the epitympanic and mastoid spaces

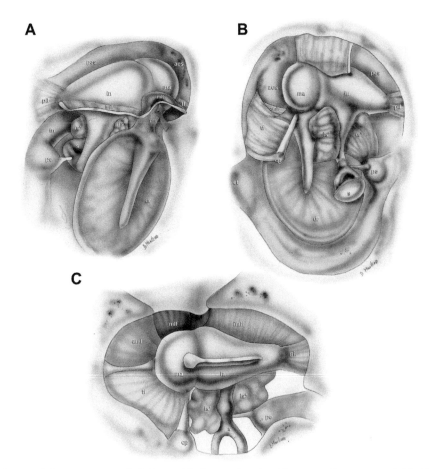

Fig. 4. Right ear. Tympanic isthmus block associated with a complete tensor fold. The blockage of the attic aeration pathway could create a selective negative pressure in the atticomastoid spaces, developing a selective retraction in the attic. Transcanal view (*A*); medial to lateral view (*B*); axial view at the level of the attic (*C*). aes, anterior epitympanic compartment; amf, anterior malleal fold; cp, cochleariform process; dr, eardrum; et, eustachian tube; fn, facial nerve; imlf, lateral incudomalleal fold; in, incus; is*, isthmus blockage; ma, malleus; mlf, lateral malleal fold; pe, pyramidal eminence; pes, posterior epitympanic compartment; pil, posterior incudal ligaments; prs, Prussak space; s, stapes; tf, tensor fold.

In our series, tensor fold removal in association with a restoration of the isthmus function prevented postoperative retraction or cholesteatoma recurrence 1 year after the primary surgery. The use of the endoscope during surgery also permitted a good view of the tensor fold area and the isthmus timpani and, consequently, enabled us to understand the type of dysventilation pattern. The goal of surgery in this kind of disorder could be restoration of normal ventilation of the attical-mastoid area. This solution is possible by removing the tensor fold and restoring the functionality of the isthmus.

We recently published another study of middle ear anatomy, focusing on middle ear folds in patients with attical retractions or cholesteatoma and with a normal tubal function test, who underwent endoscopic surgery. This scenario might describe a selective

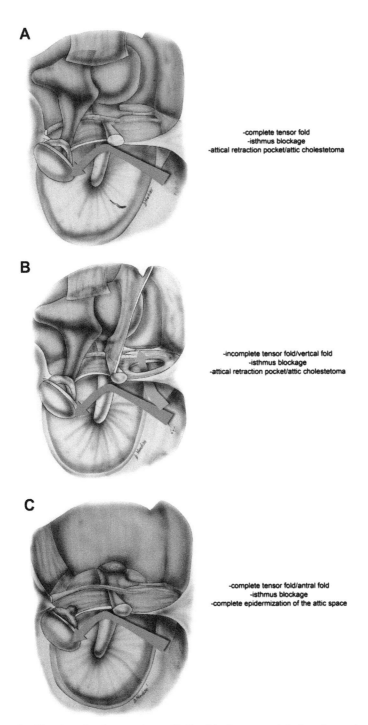

Fig. 5. Classification of epitympanic ventilation blockage correlated on the endoscopic findings. Left ear view, from medial to lateral.

epitympanic dysventilation syndrome, possibly not related to ET impairment.[8] Based on the emerging data obtained from our publications, we hypothesize a selective epitympanic dysventilation syndrome (**Fig. 6**).[10] If an isthmus blockage occurs in an ear with complete tensor and incudomalleal folds, a selective epitympanic dysventilation may manifest even with a functioning ET. The syndrome would therefore occur with the contemporaneous presence of 4 conditions: an attic retraction pocket or attic cholesteatoma, a type A tympanogram or a normal tubal function test, complete epitympanic diaphragm, and isthmus blockage.

In clinical practice, it is common to find an isolated retraction pocket of the pars flaccida and/or a attic cholesteatoma, limited to the epitympanum, with an otherwise normal pars tensa and mesotympanum. As confirmed during surgery, an open ET and a good protympanic mucosa appearance were found in cases of selective dysventilation.

To treat this condition, and perhaps to prevent cholesteatoma formation, a surgery of the isthmus should be done restoring the ventilation pathway through this anatomical structure and a new ventilation route should be created during surgery, and this can be performed by endoscopic middle ear surgery in a preservative way.

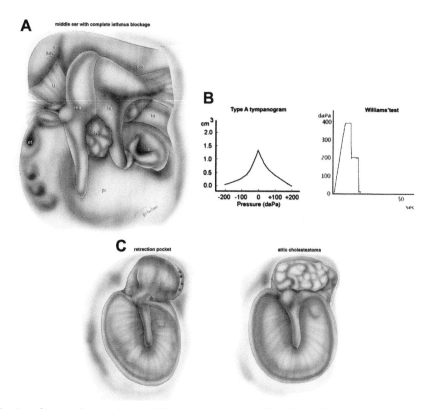

Fig. 6. Left ear. Selective dysventilation syndrome. To define this syndrome, 3 conditions are necessary: attic retraction pocket or cholesteatoma (*C*); type A tympanogram or a William test positive for a normal function of eustachian tube (*B*); complete epitympanic diaphragm associated with block of the isthmus (*A*). aes, anterior epitympanic compartment; et, eustachian tube; fn, facial nerve; in, incus; is, isthmus blockage; ma, malleus; pes, posterior epitympanic compartment; s, stapes; tf, tensor fold.

From this point of view, we suggest that, during middle ear surgery, special attention is paid to restoring an isthmus ventilation pathway, removing inflammatory tissue, or creating a new isthmus with an ossiculoplasty; the tensor fold usually should be removed to create an accessory ventilation route to the epitympanum. The aforementioned procedures are necessary for good epitympanic ventilation. Awareness and early diagnosis of selective middle ear dysventilation problems in the future could prevent the development of chronic otitis and cholesteatoma.

In another recent study,[15] we described 3 main types of endoscopic tympanoplasty that can be performed for surgical treatment of attic retraction pockets, preserving the ventilation routes, physiology, and anatomy of the middle ear as much as possible. When the disease is located in the tympanic cavity without mastoid involvement, the exclusive transcanal endoscopic approach was indicated to eradicate the disease, preserving the mastoid function and restoring the ventilation routes of the middle ear.

When an isthmus blockage was present with a normal ossicular chain, the disease was carefully removed from the isthmus by dissecting the pathologic tissue from the incudostapedial joint and the cochleariform process, and restoring ventilation through the isthmus without disrupting the chain. When the tensor fold was complete, the fold was removed, creating a direct communication from the protympanum to the anterior epitympanic space; this surgical procedure was classified as tympanolpasty type 1.

When the retraction pocket is in the superior portions of the epitympanic compartment and it is not completely visible with the endoscope, removal of part of the scutum

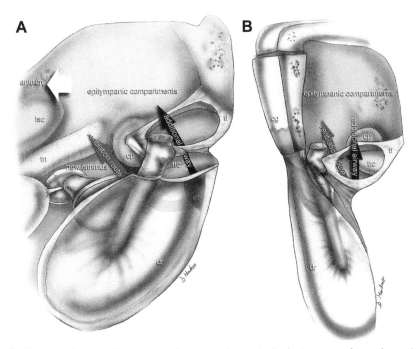

Fig. 7. Right ear. Endoscopic tympanoplasty type 2: a ossiculoplasty was performed creating a new functional isthmus (*red arrow* the main ventilation route from the ET to the attic) and the tensor fold was removed creating an additional aeration pathway from the ET to the Attic (*blue arrow*), Panel A: from later to medial view; Panel B: anterior view. cg, cartilage graft; cp, cochleariform process; dr, eardrum; fn, facial nerve; lsc, lateral semicircular canal; tf, tensor fold; ttc, tensor tendon canal.

is necessary and a wide atticotomy should be performed. A tragal graft has been used to reconstruct small defects, whereas a segment of mastoid cortical bone has been used to reconstruct larger scutum defects.

In patients with an attical aeration pattern with erosion of the ossicular chain or in subjects in whom erosion of the incus is present with disruption of the incudostapedial joint associated with blockage of the isthmus an Endoscopic tympanoplasty type 2 is attempted, new isthmus was created with a lower ossiculoplasty and the head of the malleus was cut, creating a wide and well-ventilated epitympanic compartment. When an isthmus blockage was present with erosion of the long process of the incus, a lower ossiculoplasty was performed with a remodeled incus placed on the stapes. In this way, it was possible to create a new wide isthmus, the tensor fold was removed, creating a direct communication between the protympanum and the anterior epitympanic space and permitting an additional aeration pathway (**Fig. 7**).

In some cases, a complete epidermization of the attical and the antrum region was present, and it was not possible to restore good ventilation in the epitympanic compartments because of the high risk of residual cholesteatoma. What might be termed an endoscopic open technique was performed (Tympanoplasty type 3), excluding the epitympanic compartment from the tympanic cavity by temporalis fascia interposition; the tympanic cavity was excluded from the epitympanum by a complete lateral attic bony wall removal and with interposition of the temporalis fascia in the antrum. This approach allowed us to create ventilation of the middle ear, excluding the mastoid and the epitympanum from the tympanic cavity. In this way, tympanoplasty tensor fold resection was not required because fascia was placed over the tensor fold.

SUMMARY

The physiopathology of middle ear disease requires proper understanding, and endoscopic middle ear surgery may help provide this, allowing the surgeon to explore all ventilation pathways without radically changing middle ear anatomy. In this way, the surgical approach must be the focused. The restoration of an adequate ventilation route between the mesotympanum and epitympanum, and, in our experience, surgical treatment of attic retraction or cholesteatoma limited to the tympanic cavity, can be achieved exclusively by the endoscopic approach.

REFERENCES

1. Prussak A. Zur Anatomie des menschlichen Trommelfells. Arch Ohrenheilkd 1867;3:255–78.
2. Palva T, Johnsson L. Epitympanic compartment surgical considerations: reevaluation. Am J Otol 1995;16:505–13.
3. Lin AC, Messner AH. Pediatric tympanoplasty: factors affecting success. Curr Opin Otolaryngol Head Neck Surg 2008;16:64–8.
4. Marchioni D, Mattioli F, Alicandri-Ciufelli M, et al. Endoscopic evaluation of middle ear ventilation route blockage. Am J Otolaryngol 2010;31(6):453–66.
5. Lemoine J. The role of interattico-tympanic diaphragm in the pathogenesis of otitis in infants, Nourrisson 1950;38(1):1–64.
6. Proctor B. The development of the middle ear spaces and their surgical significance. J Laryngol Otol 1964;78:631–48.
7. Marchioni D, Alicandri-Ciufelli M, Grammatica A, et al. Lateral endoscopic approach to epitympanic diaphragm and Prussak's space: a dissection study. Surg Radiol Anat 2010;32(9):843–52.

8. Marchioni D, Alicandri-Ciufelli M, Molteni G, et al. Selective epitympanic dysventilation syndrome. Laryngoscope 2010;120(5):1028–33.

9. Palva T, Ramsay H, Bohling T. Tensor fold and anterior epitympanum. Am J Otol 1997;18:307–16.

10. Marchioni D, Grammatica A, Alicandri-Ciufelli M. The contribution of selective dysventilation to attical middle ear pathology. Med Hypotheses 2011;77(1): 116–20.

11. Marchioni D, Mattioli F, Alicandri-Ciufelli M, et al. Endoscopic approach to tensor fold in patients with attic cholesteatoma. Acta Otolaryngol 2009;129(9):946–54.

12. Marchioni D, Mattioli F, Cobelli M, et al. CT morphological evaluation of anterior epitympanic recess in patients with attic cholesteatoma. Eur Arch Otorhinolaryngol 2008;12:12–3.

13. Tanabe M, Takahashi H, Honjo I, et al. Gas exchange function of middle ear in patients with otitis media with effusion. Eur Arch Otorhinolaryngol 1997;254: 453–5.

14. Gorur K, Ozcan C, Talas DU. The computed tomographical and tympanometrical evaluation of mastoid pneumatization and attic blockage in patients with chronic otitis media with effusion. Int J Pediatr Otorhinolaryngol 2006;70:481–5.

15. Marchioni D, Alicandri-Ciufelli M, Molteni G, et al. Endoscopic tympanoplasty in patients with attic retraction pockets. Laryngoscope 2010;120(9):1847–55.

Endoscopic Anatomy of the Retrotympanum

João Flávio Nogueira, MD[a],*, Francesco Mattioli, MD[b],
Livio Presutti, MD[b], Daniele Marchioni, MD[b]

KEYWORDS

- Surgical anatomy • Cholesteatoma • Middle ear • Retrotympanum • Atraumatic

KEY POINTS

- The retrotympanum is located at the posterior portion and houses several important and complex anatomic and surgical structures.
- The greater the depth of the subpyramidal space (SS), the more is a surgical approach at high risk of leaving residual cholesteatoma.
- Use of the endoscope in the middle ear recesses in cholesteatoma surgery may reduce the residual cholesteatoma rate. Using a transcanal minimally invasive approach allows the preservation of bone and mucosa of the mastoid cell system. This atraumatic approach is a suitable method for exploring the mesotympanic structures.
- In type C sinus tympani (ST), especially associated with a well-developed mastoid cell system, it is not always possible to have a good control of the ST using endoscopes; in these cases, a combined (endoscopic-microscopic) posterior retrofacial approach is suggested.

ANATOMY OF RETROTYMPANUM

The middle ear can be divided into subspaces, based on their relationship with the mesotympanum. Superior to it lies the epitympanum; anterior to it, the protympanum; and inferior to it, the hypotympanum.[1]

The retrotympanum is located at the posterior portion and houses several important and complex anatomic and surgical structures. Its anatomy represents a challenge both in understanding and visualization, because conventional transcanal microscopic approaches can neither visualize nor preserve some of those important structures.[1,2] Recently, endoscopic techniques have allowed the complete visualization of these structures.

This article describes the endoscopic anatomy of the retrotympanum and its relationships to other important anatomic landmarks in the middle ear to understand its importance and relevance during surgical procedures.

[a] UECE – State University of Ceara, Fortaleza, Brazil; [b] ENT Department, University Hospital of Modena, Via del Pozzo 71, Modena, Italy
* Corresponding author.
E-mail address: joaoflavioce@hotmail.com

Otolaryngol Clin N Am 46 (2013) 179–188
http://dx.doi.org/10.1016/j.otc.2012.10.003
oto.theclinics.com

The retrotympanum is divided by the subiculum into superior and inferior retrotympanum. The superior retrotympanum can also be subdivided in 4 spaces: 2 medially and anteriorly and 2 laterally and posteriorly to the third tract of facial nerve.[1,2]

The ST is one of the most important spaces of the retrotympanum. It is represented by[1–4]

- Posterior outpouching cavity lying between the medial wall of the middle ear medially
- The pyramidal eminence (PE) laterally
- Posterolateral delineation by the second genu and third tract of the facial nerve, lateral semicircular canal (LSC), and vestibule
- Close relationship anteriorly with the superior portion of the promontory

The ST is bordered superiorly by the ponticulus that separates it from the posterior tympanic sinus (PTS), a bone niche of the superior portion of the retrotympanum.

PTS is not always present, depending on the presence of ponticulus and the extension of ST, by the oval window, and inferiorly by the subiculum, that separates it from the inferior retrotympanum and round window. This space could also be divided into 3 different types depending on its posterior extension with respect of the third portion of the facial nerve. Laterally and posteriorly to the second genu and vertical portion of the seventh cranial nerve are localized 2 anatomic bone niches: the facial sinus and the lateral tympanic sinus. These niches are separated by the chordal ridge, departing from the posterior portion of the PE. These anatomic regions are more accessible than ST and PTS because they are located laterally to a tangential plane passing on the seventh cranial nerve course, and their anatomies are more constant.[1–6]

The PE is a triangular bony structure, with its base oriented posteriorly and the tip anteriorly. The PE houses the stapes tendon and has a horizontal orientation, lying anteriorly and laterally to the second genu of the facial nerve.[3,4]

Under this bone structure, that is located at the middle of retrotympanum, is the SS, which is delimited laterally by the medial aspect of the PE, medially by the medial side of the bony wall of the retrotympanum, and posteriorly by the vertical tract of the seventh cranial nerve.

This space can present different morphologies, mostly in its depth, varying from a total absence, because of total ossification of the medial aspect of the PE with the medial wall of retrotympanum, to a particularly deep SS lying beneath the facial nerve.

The inferior retrotympanum is the posterior space that houses the sinus subtympanicus (SSt), delimited posteriorly by the styloid complex and the third portion of the seventh cranial nerve; anteriorly by the round window with its pillars, tegmen, and the inferior and posterior portions of the promontory; superiorly by the subiculum; and inferiorly by the jugular bulb.[1–6]

Endoscopic Anatomy of the Retrotympanum

Recent endoscopic anatomy study[7] clearly describes the following ST shape variations:

a. *Classical shape*: when the sinus is located between the ponticulus and subiculum, lying medial to the facial nerve and to the pyramidal process (**Fig. 1**A)
b. *Confluent shape*: when an incomplete ponticulus is present and the ST is confluent to the posterior sinus (see **Fig. 1**B)
c. *Partitioned shape*: when a ridge of bone extending from the third portion of the facial nerve to the promontory area is present, separating the ST into 2 portions (superior and inferior) (see **Fig. 1**C)

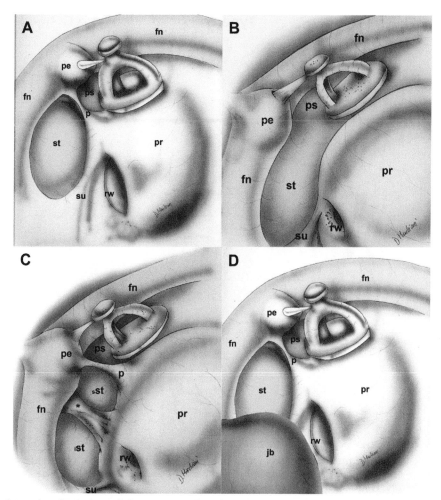

Fig. 1. (*A–D*)Drawing of the anatomy describing the sinus tympani shape variations. fn, facial nerve; jb, jugular bulb; p, ponticulum; pe, pyramidal eminence; pr, promontory; ps, posterior sinus; rw, round window; su, subiculum; st, sinus tympani.

d. *Restricted shape*: when a high jugular bulb is present, thus reducing the inferior extension of the ST (see **Fig. 1**D)

Several anatomic studies focused on the depth of ST. This detail is important because the greater the depth of the ST, the more is it difficult to achieve the complete removal of cholesteatoma, especially using traditional microscopic approaches. This is particularly true when the ST is deep. For this reason, it might be useful for the surgeon to study the extension of the ST before the surgery.

Another important endoscopic anatomic study[8] classified the depth of the ST into 3 types as follows:

- *Type A*: small ST. The medial limit of the third portion of the facial nerve corresponds to the depth of the sinus. In these cases, the ST is small and does not present a medial and posterior extension to the facial nerve (**Fig. 2**).

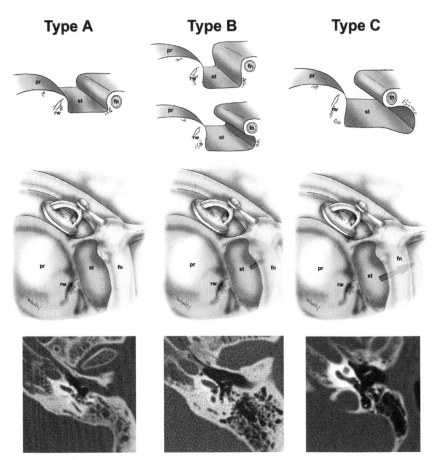

Fig. 2. Drawing of the classification of the sinus tympani depth. Red arrow indicates posterior extension of Sinus timpani respect the third portion of facial nerve. fn, facial nerve; Pr, promontory; rw, round window; st, sinus tympani.

- *Type B*: deep ST. The medial boundary of the ST lies medially with respect to the third portion of the facial nerve; however, it does not present a posterior extension to the facial nerve (see **Fig. 2**).
- *Type C*: deep ST with posterior extension. The medial boundary of the ST lies medial and posterior to the third portion of the facial nerve. In these cases, ST is very large and deep, and all these patients have a well-developed mastoid (see **Fig. 2**).

When a patient has a type C ST, it is not possible to explore the entire depth of the sinus, not even with the help of the endoscope, especially when it is associated with a well-developed mastoid cell system. In these cases, it is necessary to perform a posterior retrofacial approach.[7–9]

Endoscopic Anatomy of the Ponticulus

The endoscopic transcanal approach to the ST also permits a good view of the ponticulus. The ponticulus is a bony ridge extending from the pyramidal process to the promontory region, which separates the ST from the PTS.

Endoscopic anatomy study described the following 3 different variants of the ponticulus[7]:

a. *Classical morphology*: (**Fig. 3**A) in patients with such morphology, the ponticulus is completely formed and it is like a ridge of bone extending from the pyramidal process to the promontory area; this structure represents the superior limit of ST, dividing it from posterior sinus.
b. *Incomplete ponticulus*: (see **Fig. 3**B) in this morphology, the ST and posterior sinus are confluent.
c. *Communicating ponticulus*: in subjects with this morphology, the ponticulus is like a small bridge of bone and there is a communication between the ST and the posterior sinus under it (see **Fig. 3**C).

Especially when the ponticulus is like a small bridge, intraoperative endoscopic evaluation of the ponticulus area is very useful, because a residual cholesteatoma could be present under this bony bridge.[7–11]

Endoscopic Anatomy of Subiculum

The endoscopic approach to the ST also permits a good view of the subiculum.[7,8] Subiculum is a bony ridge extending outward from the posterior tip of the round window niche to the styloid eminence region, which separates the ST from the SSt.

When the subiculum is present, ST is separated by inferior retrotympanum (**Fig. 4**); when the subiculum is absent, the ST is confluent to the inferior retrotympanum.

The bridge subiculum is a rare conformation. When present, under this bridge of bone there is a communication between the inferior retrotympanum and the ST.

Endoscopic Anatomy of Subpyramidal Space

Endoscopic anatomy study[7,8] also describes close and variable relationships between ST, PTS, and the PE. Pneumatization of the retrotympanum may extend to a variable degree into a recess under the PE. This region is called the SS.

This space is limited laterally by the medial aspect of the pyramidal process, medially by the lateral wall of the tympanum, inferiorly by the ponticulus, and posteriorly and superiorly by the Fallopian canal, and it could be in direct anatomic continuity with the ST or with the PTS, depending on the position of the ponticulus. Features of this space (particularly its depth) vary significantly, and the authors have observed that it could range from total absence, due to the complete development of the medial aspect of the pyramidal process, to a clear representation of the SS with a significant depth. When the medial face of the PE is completely formed, the SS is large and

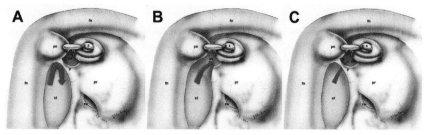

Fig. 3. (*A–C*) Drawing showing different types of ponticulus. Red arrow indicates represents the sinus tympani shape. fn, facial nerve; p, ponticulum; pe, pyramidal eminence; pr, promontory; ps, posterior sinus; rw, round window; st, sinus tympani.

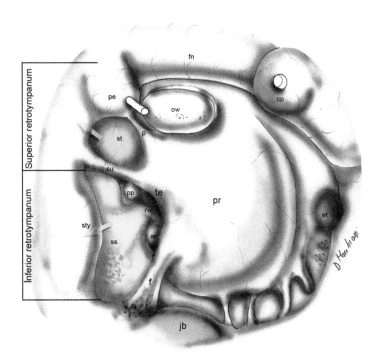

Fig. 4. Anatomy of subiculum. Yellow arrow indicates the depth of SS e ST. ap, anterior pillar; cp, cochleariform process; et, Eustachian tube; f, finiculus; fn, facial nerve; jb, jugular bulb; p, ponticulum; pe, pyramidal eminence; pp, posterior pillar; pr, promontory; ss, sinus subtimpanicum; st, sinus tympani; su, subiculum; rw, round window.

bounded by both the ST and PTS (*independent morphology of the PE*), and when the medial face of the PE is partially formed (*partial morphology of the PE*), the SS is narrow and in some cases very deep, thus the posterior extension of this space is not explorable with an endoscope (**Fig. 5**).

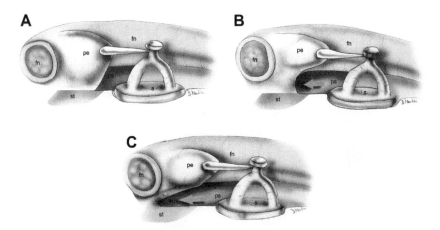

Fig. 5. (*A–C*) Anatomic variations of the subpyramidal space. Yellow arrow indicates the depth of PE. fn, facial nerve; pe, pyramidal eminence; ps, posterior sinus; st, sinus tympani; ps, pyramidal space.

In some cases that the authors observed, the medial bony wall of the PE was absent and the eminence was completely merged with the medial bone of the retrotympanum; in this case, the SS was not present *(merged morphology of the PE)* (see **Fig. 5**A).

The greater the depth of SS, the more is a surgical approach at high risk of leaving residual cholesteatoma. Thus, a good knowledge of these anatomic spaces may help in reducing the risk of residual cholesteatoma during middle ear surgery.[9–11]

Endoscopic Anatomy of Inferior Retrotympanum

Although surgeons have already studied the anatomy of the inferior retrotympanum,[1–5] this region has been quite neglected in the literature, most likely due to the low accessibility of this space during conventional microscopic procedures. In fact, in their studies, Proctor and colleagues have already identified almost all the structures in this region based on several temporal bone dissections.[12]

Proctor identified a quite constant structure, a ridge of bone connecting the basal helix of the cochlea to the jugular wall of the tympanum, in relation to the anterior pillar of the round window niche: the *sustentaculum promontorii*.

He called it the *sustentaculum* (from the Latin *sustentaculum, -i*: support) because he thought that it sustained the inferior tympanic artery, enveloping it during the development of the middle ear. Marchioni and colleagues[7,8] confirmed the presence of this structure in relation to the anterior pillar of the round niche, identifying 2 variants: a ridge shape and a bridge shape. They[7,8] decided to rename the sustentaculum promontorii as the *finiculus* for the following reasons:

- It is quite unlikely that the inferior tympanic artery constantly lies in this structure, particularly in the case of the bridge shape, because it could be a very thin structure in some cases.
- Moreover, the authors wanted to identify a clear borderline between the retrotympanum and the hypotympanum, and for this they chose to rename it finiculus (from the Latin *finis, -is*: borderline). This anatomic structure can have some different conformations (**Figs. 6** and **7**).

Proctor also defined a bony structure, representing a kind of floor of the retrotympanic region, that he called the area concamerata. Although the pars media of the area concamerata (Proctor's "fustis"), a smooth bony column mainly forming the floor of the round window niche, can be easily identified in some of our ears, the authors found it somewhat difficult to identify the other parts of the area concamerata.

Marchioni noticed that in several patients a sinus lying inferior to the ST could be identified, forming a well-delimited space between the subiculum superiorly and posteriorly and the finiculus inferiorly and anteriorly, limited posteriorly and laterally by the styloid eminence and posteriorly and medially by otic capsule, and open anteriorly and medially to the round window niche. Marchioni called this space the "sinus subtympanicus."

ANATOMIC IMPORTANCE

When the cholesteatoma involves the ST, there might be 2 clinically important risks. One is the potential for residual disease because of incomplete removal of the disease, and the second is the increased risk for ossicular discontinuity and hearing loss because of cholesteatoma within the ST, which the surgeon cannot control.[13,14]

To avoid these risks, maximum exposure of the ST and complete removal of the disease are essential. However, the ST remains a challenging location in cholesteatoma surgery because it is made relatively inaccessible by the facial nerve and the stapedial muscle and tendon, when using microscopic traditional approaches,

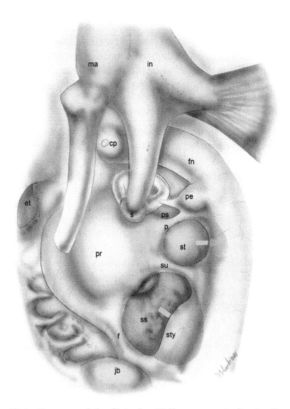

Fig. 6. Anatomy. Note the area of the finiculus. Yellow arrow indicates the depth of SS e ST. cp, cochleariform process; et, Eustachian tube; f, finiculus; fn, facial nerve; in, incus; jb, jugular bulb; Ma, malleolus; p, ponticulus; pe, pyramidal eminence; ps, posterior sinus; s, stapes; ss, sinus subtimpanicum; st, sinus tympani; sty, styloid process; su, subiculum.

because of the inherent limitations of this instrument. For this reason, the surgical management of ST cholesteatoma remains controversial. Residual cholesteatoma is among the major causes of failure in surgical treatment of cholesteatoma.[15–17]

Residual cholesteatoma occurs as a consequence of growth of a fragment of the matrix inadvertently remaining in the middle ear at the time of cholesteatoma surgery.

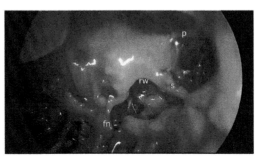

Fig. 7. Endoscopic anatomy showing the finiculus (fn), ponticulum (p), round window niche (rw), and subiculum (s).

Some investigators focused on the frequency of residual cholesteatoma detected with the intraoperative use of the endoscope after traditional microscopic surgery.[18,19] They found that the ST was the most common site of residual cholesteatoma fragments.

The problems of residual cholesteatoma depend on the surgical approach; in fact, poor access cannot permit accurate cholesteatoma removal. For this reason, the particular anatomy of the ST requires maximum surgical exposure to permit complete removal of the disease. Several surgical techniques have been described to approach the ST area, all with the help of an operative microscope.[15–17]

Recently, a posterior approach to the ST through the mastoid was proposed by several investigators.[3] The retrofacial posterior approach was performed by dissecting the triangular bony area formed by the facial nerve, LSC, and posterior semicircular canal. This approach is very difficult and requires an expert otologic surgeon because the facial nerve, the posterior semicircular canal, and the LSC are all at risk of injury.

However, the development of endoscopic techniques for the middle ear has permitted exploration of hidden recesses such as the ST. Thomassin and colleagues[19–23] found that the quality of disease eradication had significantly improved with the intraoperative use of the endoscope, which allowed a consequent reduction of residual cholesteatoma.

Using the endoscope in the middle ear recesses in cholesteatoma surgery, we may reduce the residual cholesteatoma rate, using a transcanal minimally invasive approach that allows the preservation of bone and mucosa of the mastoid cell system, which have an important functional role at the middle ear homeostasis. This atraumatic approach is a suitable method for exploring the mesotympanic structures.

The literature[7,8] presents clear description of the endoscopic approaches to retrotympanum (with 0°, 45°, and 70° optics); these approaches ensure the complete visualization of the retrotympanum surgical spaces, and these techniques may allow the surgeon to completely visualize the anatomic variations and pathologic tissues. The transcanal endoscopic approach to the ST is indicated in ST of types A and B. When the surgical field is bleeding extensively, it is often necessary to clean the optical instruments and, in some cases, the surgeon must change the approach. In type C ST, especially associated with a well-developed mastoid cell system, it is not always possible to have good control of the ST using endoscopes; in these cases, a combined (endoscopic-microscopic) posterior retrofacial approach is suggested.[7–9]

Advantages of Endoscopic Approach

Endoscopic approach to ST and retrotympanum offers a direct mini-invasive surgical approach to the middle ear avoiding mastoid bone and mucosa removal. Also, it allows a direct visualization of the retrotympanum and surrounding structures such as ossicular chain, chorda tympani, facial nerve, and round and oval window niches, offering a wide exposition of the retrotympanic region both medially (ST, sinus subtympanicus, subpyramidal space) and laterally (facial sinus, lateral sinus).

REFERENCES

1. Donaldson JA, Anson BJ, Warphea RL, et al. The surgical anatomy of the sinus tympani. Arch Otolaryngol 1970;91:219–27.
2. Baki FA, El Dine MB, El Said L, et al. Sinus tympani endoscopic anatomy. Otolaryngol Head Neck Surg 2002;127:158–62.
3. Pickett BP, Cail WS, Lambert PR. Sinus tympani: anatomic considerations, computed tomography, and a discussion of the retrofacial approach for removal of disease. Am J Otol 1995;16:541–50.

4. Ozturan O, Bauer CA, Miller CC, et al. Dimensions of the sinus tympani and its surgical access via a retrofacial approach. Ann Otol Rhinol Laryngol 1996;105: 776–83.
5. Steinbrugge H. On sinus tympani. Arch Otolaryngol 1889;8:53–7.
6. Holt JJ. The ponticulus: an anatomic study. Otol Neurotol 2005;26:1122–4.
7. Marchioni D, Alicandri-Ciufelli M, Piccinini A, et al. Inferior retrotympanum revisited: an endoscopic anatomic study. Laryngoscope 2010;120(9):1880–6.
8. Marchioni D, Mattioli F, Alicandri-Ciufelli M, et al. Transcanal endoscopic approach to the sinus tympani: a clinical report. Otol Neurotol 2009;30(6):758–65.
9. Presutti L, Marchioni D, Mattioli F, et al. Endoscopic management of acquired cholesteatoma: our experience. J Otolaryngol 2008;4:1–7.
10. Badr-El-Dine M. Value of ear endoscopy in cholesteatoma surgery. Otol Neurotol 2002;23:631–5.
11. Tarabichi M. Endoscopic management of acquired cholesteatoma. Am J Otol 1997;18:544–9.
12. Proctor B. The development of the middle ear spaces and their surgical significance. J Laryngol Otol 1964;78:631–48.
13. Weiss MH, Parisier SC, Han JC, et al. Surgery for recurrent and residual cholesteatoma. Laryngoscope 1992;102:145–51.
14. Jeng FC, Tsai MH, Brown CJ. Relationship of preoperative findings and ossicular discontinuity in chronic otitis media. Otol Neurotol 2003;24:29–32.
15. Pulec JL. Sinus tympani: retrofacial approach for the removal of cholesteatomas. Ear Nose Throat J 1996;75:77–88.
16. Farrior JB. Tympanoplasty: the anterior attico-tympanotomy. Surgery of the posterior tympanic recess. Laryngoscope 1968;78:768–79.
17. Goodhill V. Circumferential tympanomastoid access: the sinus tympani area. Ann Otol Rhinol Laryngol 1973;82:547–54.
18. El-Meselaty K, Badr-El-Dine M, Mandour M, et al. Endoscope affects decision making in cholesteatoma surgery. Otolaryngol Head Neck Surg 2003;129:490–6.
19. Thomassin JM, Korchia D, Doris JM. Endoscopic guided otosurgery in the prevention of residual cholesteatomas. Laryngoscope 1993;103:939–43.
20. Tarabichi M. Endoscopic management of limited attic cholesteatoma. Laryngoscope 2004;114:1157–62.
21. Bowdler DA, Walsh RM. Comparison of the otoendoscopic and microscopic anatomy of the middle ear cleft in canal wall-up and canal wall-down temporal bone dissections. Clin Otolaryngol Allied Sci 1995;20:418–22.
22. Bottril ID, Poe DS. Endoscope-assisted ear surgery. Am J Otol 1995;16:158–63.
23. Karhuketo TS, Puhakka HJ, Laippala PJ. Endoscopy of the middle ear structures. Acta Otolaryngol Suppl 1997;529:34–9.

Beyond the Middle Ear
Endoscopic Surgical Anatomy and Approaches to Inner Ear and Lateral Skull Base

Livio Presutti, MD[a],*, João Flávio Nogueira, MD[b],
Matteo Alicandri-Ciufelli, MD[a], Daniele Marchioni, MD[a]

KEYWORDS

- Transcanal endoscopic approach • Petrous bone pathologic condition
- Lateral skull base • Surgical anatomy • Inner ear

KEY POINTS

- The endoscopic approach to lateral skull base can be classified as a transcanal exclusively endoscopic approach or as combined approaches (microscopic endoscope-assisted): transotic, infralabyrinthine, and suprameatal translabyrinthine.
- The transcanal exclusive endoscopic approach allows eradication of pathologic conditions involving the petrous apex, internal ear canal fundus, with extension limited to the intracochlear, intravestibular, and pericartoid regions. If the pathologic state involves the mastoid, an exclusive approach is not feasible.
- The transotic endoscope-assisted approach allows the removal of big lesions, which completely involve the petrous bone, with hearing loss compromised (ie, cholesterol granulomas). In particular, endoscope introduction is indicated for the control of the paraclival region and for the control of the carotid artery at the level of the clivus and the petrous apex.
- The infralabyrinthine endoscope-assisted approach is indicated for lesions extending inferiorly to the labyrinth. This approach allows removal of pathologic matter without loss of hearing.
- The suprameatal translabirinthine endoscope-assisted approach is indicated for pathologic conditions (mainly cholesteatomas) involving the labyrinthine tract of the facial nerve with or without internal auditory canal extension facial nerve tract with or without internal auditory canal extension.

All the authors have read and approved the manuscript. The authors have no financial relationship to disclose.
 ^a Otolaryngology Department, University Hospital of Modena, Via del Pozzo 71, Modena 41100, Italy; ^b Instituto de Otorrinolaringologia e Oftalmologia de Fortaleza - IOF Sinus Centro, Fortaleza, Ceara, Brazil
* Corresponding author.
E-mail address: presutti.livio@policlinico.mo.it

INTRODUCTION

Endoscopic instrumentation, techniques, and knowledge have improved during the last few years and the authors believe that, in the future, endoscopic surgical techniques will gain increasing importance in otologic surgery. The authors' experience in endoscopic ear surgery leads to the belief that most of the spaces considered to be difficult to access with the microscopic technique could be easily visualized by endoscope-assisted surgery or by exclusively endoscopic approaches.[1,2] Moreover, the authors think that new anatomic,[1] physiologic,[3,4] and surgical concepts[1,5–8] should be introduced for this purpose.

A gradual introduction of endoscopic techniques to treatment of pathologic conditions of the middle ear began in the 1990s.[9] Endoscopies were primarily used for the visualization of hidden areas such as the posterior epitympanum during classic microscopic tympanoplasty.[10] Gradually, endoscopies were used also in an operative fashion, to substitute for the microscope as a main tool during middle ear operations.[2,7,8] At present, the main application of endoscopic surgery is in middle ear cholesteatoma surgery but, in the natural evolution of the technique, there are the steps forward of lateral skull base surgery. In recent years, the authors began to notice that the internal ear and the whole temporal bone could be accessed in an endoscopic-assisted fashion or by an exclusive endoscopic approach. The only problem would be codifying, as much as possible, the landmarks and the procedures, and integrating them to classic microscopic approaches. At present some experiences of endoscopic ear surgery of the lateral skull base have already been made, both on cadaver dissection and in living patients. The codification of the initial exclusively endoscopic approaches was based on cadavers. The first steps of the procedures were attempted for cholesteatoma treatment or for exploration and study of middle ear. The codification of the endoscopic approaches in combination with microscopic approaches come, on the other hand, from clinical experiences in which endoscopes were used as an aid for microscopic-based approaches to internal ear or petrous treatment of pathologic conditions of bone.

Summarizing these concepts, the approaches can be classified as follows:

A. Transcanal exclusively endoscopic approach
B. Combined approaches: microscopic endoscope-assisted
   - Intralabyrinthine (**Fig. 1**A)
   - Suprameatal translabyrinthine (see **Fig. 1**B)
   - Transotic (see **Fig. 1**C).

The aim of this article is to analyze the morphology and surgical and anatomic findings of the approach to lateral skull base surgery, petrous apex, internal ear, and internal auditory canal by using exclusive or combined endoscopic techniques.

TRANSCANAL EXCLUSIVE ENDOSCOPIC APPROACH

This endoscopic approach allows eradication of pathologic matter involving petrous apex, internal ear canal fundus, with extension limited to the intracochlear, intravestibular, and pericartoid regions. If the pathologic condition involves the mastoid, an exclusive approach is not feasible.

Possible indications are

   - Mesotympanic cholesteatomas with medial extension toward inner ear structures
   - Cholesterol granulomas of the petrous apex

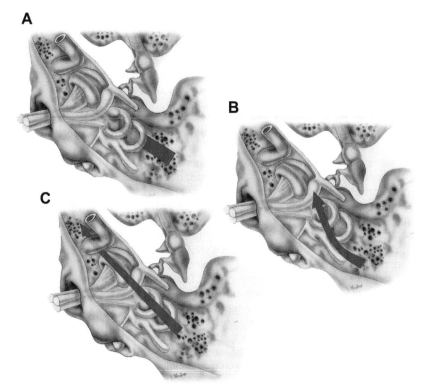

Fig. 1. (*Left ear*) The combined approaches to the inner ear. Arrows indicate direction of procedures. (*A*) Infralabyrinthine. (*B*) Suprameatal translabyrinthine. (*C*) Transotic.

- Small symptomatic or growing acoustic neuromas with exclusive extension to internal ear canal fundus
- Cochlear schwannomas with or without internal ear canal fundus extension
- Facial nerve schwannomas involving timpani tract and geniculate ganglion.

Clinical application of this approach is currently limited, although preliminary experiences and results following initial attempts are promising. Even indications for surgery in some of the pathologic conditions treated by these approaches could change in the future as a result of these minimally invasive operations, compared with the extensive bony tissue removal that microscopic techniques require.

Preliminary Surgical Steps

Using a transcanal endoscopic approach, a circumferential incision of the external ear canal skin is made approximately 3 cm from the annulus by a 0° degree endoscope.

Tympanic membrane and external ear canal skin are then removed en bloc to obtain the widest exposition of the middle ear. Using a 0° degree endoscope, a circumferential drilling is made to further increase the view and to facilitate maneuvering of surgical instruments.

Next, it is fundamental to identify the great vessels that have close relationships to the middle ear (ie, the jugular bulb and carotid artery). The first is found at the level of hypotympanum and the second at the level of protympanum, close to the eustachian tube. In some cases, an extensive drilling at those levels are required, in other cases the vessels are clearly identified without drilling any bony tissue.

Next, the incus and the malleus are removed. This allows the surgeon better access to the tympani tract of the facial nerve, to the geniculate ganglion region, and to the greater petrosal nerve, which is located anteriorly.[6]

The tympanic tract of the facial nerve and the greater petrosal nerve are then skeletonized. The cochleariform process should be removed, uncovering the underlying tensor tympani muscle. This step could be performed in a posterior to anterior direction using a microcurette because the bone at this level is very thin. In some cases the muscle need to be cauterized due to the bleeding that these procedures might provoke. When cauterizing, pay attention to the proximity of the geniculate ganglion at this level.

Once the tensor tympani canal has been removed, dissection of the muscle itself is done, displacing it anteriorly. In this way an adequate space is achieved to enable surgery directed to the geniculate ganglion and greater petrosal nerve. The relationship between the superior and lateral border of the tensor tympani canal and the facial nerve (in particular the geniculate ganglion in its posterior and inferior aspect) is apparent.

If the pathologic matter extends anteriorly to the pericartoid region, an increased skeletonization of the greater petrosal nerve should be made in a posterior to anterior direction, by also identifying the dura of the middle cranial fossa, which at this level is situated very close to the geniculate ganglion. The greater petrosal nerve represents a fundamental landmark for this procedure because it has an almost parallel course to the horizontal tract of the carotid artery.

If the lesion has an intracochlear or intravestibular extension with or without extension to the fundus of internal ear canal, the identification of the labyrinthine tract of the facial nerve should be performed. The nerve should be followed from geniculate ganglion to its entry into the internal auditory canal with either a transvestibular or a transcochlear approach.

The choice of the approach will depend on which lesion is being removed and, in particular, will depend on the internal auditory canal involvement and the bone erosion provoked by the pathologic state.

TRANSVESTIBULAR APPROACH

A transvestibular approach is indicated in cases of lesions from the tympanic cavity that cause a wide erosion of the cochlea and vestibule, creating communication with the internal ear canal fundus, and lesions coming from the internal auditory canal fundus with or without cochlear involvement (eg, small acoustic neuromas from the fundus or cochlear schwannomas). The stapes is removed from the oval window to expose the internal ear spaces at this level. The oval window is enlarged in a anterior and inferior direction to obtain a good exposition of the medial aspect of the bony labyrinth. The saccular fossa is identified, with the spherical recess, which is the site of medial termination of the inferior vestibular nerve. The spherical recess is a thin cribriform plate which separates vestibule from internal auditory canal fundus and this bony layer is removed by a microcurette. This step allows access to the internal auditory canal, with possible consequent cerebrospinal fluid (CSF) outflow.

Next, the facial nerve can be identified at the level of internal auditory canal, which lays close to the spherical recess, approximately 1 mm anteriorly and medially. The cochlear nerve lays inferiorly compared with the facial nerve, which terminates in the modiolus (**Fig. 2**). Once the intrameatal portion of the nerve have been identified, the identification of the intralabyrinthine tract of the nerve must be completed, and dissection of it is made in a anterior and superior direction following the facial nerve into the internal auditory canal to the geniculate ganglion.

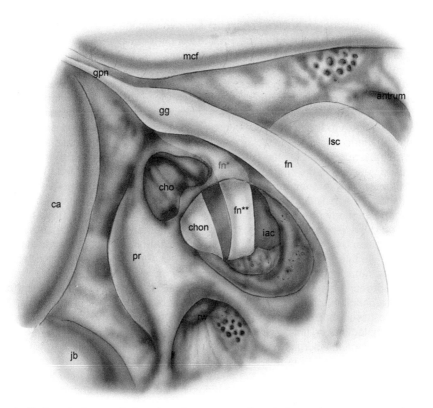

Fig. 2. (*Left ear*) The surgical cavity after transcanal exclusive endoscopic approach. ca, carotid artery; cho, cochlea; chon, cochlear nerve; fn, facial nerve; fn*, intralabyrinthine facial nerve; fn**, facial nerve on the internal auditory canal; gg, geniculate ganglion; gpn, greater petrosal nerve; iac, internal auditory canal; Jb, jugular bulb; lsc, lateral semicircular canal; mcf, middle cranial fossa; pr, promontory; rw, round window.

Before this step, identification of the middle turn of the cochlea is suggested. Because it lies close to the vestibule anteriorly, it could represent an important landmark for the identification of the intralabyrinthine tract of facial nerve, which runs just above this structure (**Fig. 2**). Another important consideration is the characteristics of the intralabyrinthine portion of the facial nerve: this tract is thin and more fragile than the other tracts of the same nerve and it is covered by a thick bony layer. For these reasons, the authors prefer to use Piezosurgery (S.R.L. medical; Mectron) dissection during those steps. The dissection substantiates following the nerve toward the internal auditory canal in an anterior and superior direction, removing the bone over the basal turn of the cochlea where the intralabyrinthine tract reaches the geniculate ganglion. Finally, the whole facial nerve can be visualized and the possible pathologic tissue can be removed while preserving the facial nerve structure.

TRANSCOCHLEAR APPROACH

The transcochlear approach has the advantage of the absence of internal auditory canal opening, avoiding CSF outflow. This approach is preferred in cases of lesions originating from the tympanic cavity, with a medial extension to the cochlea and/or vestibule without internal auditory canal fundus involvement, or of lesions originating from the timpani cavity with intracochlear and pericartoid extension, or even in cases of facial nerve schwannomas.

Nerve dissection is verified by an anatomic triangle identification between the middle turn of the cochlea, geniculate ganglion, and vestibule. The stapes is removed, followed by identification of the vestibule through the oval window. Then, a promontory drilling is made anteriorly to the vestibule and inferiorly to the geniculate ganglion. This step allows the access to the middle turn of the cochlea, which represents a landmark for the intralabyrinthine tract of the facial nerve. As mentioned above, this part of the facial nerve runs just above the cochlea, with a transverse direction from lateral to medial from geniculate ganglion to the internal auditory canal fundus. This is followed by removal, using Piezosurgery instruments, of the bony tissue laying between cochlea anteriorly and inferiorly, the geniculate ganglion anteriorly and superiorly, and the vestibule posteriorly and inferiorly (the latter representing the base of the triangle). Bone removal should be done very gently to avoid damaging to the nerve itself, which at this level is very fragile and thin. Dissection should be done carefully, to where the nerve penetrates into the internal auditory canal, trying to avoid dural tearing at this level and/or creating communications with the internal auditory canal fundus.

This approach allows the complete control of the facial nerve in its tympanic tract, geniculate ganglion, greater petrosal nerve, and labyrinthine tract of the nerve. The pathologic tissue can be removed safely and further bone removal is made based on the pathologic condition.

At the end of the surgical procedure, in case a communication with intradural spaces was created, some adipose tissue should be placed in the region of CSF leak. It is necessary to obliterate the eustachian tube and to obliterate the external auditory canal, similar to classic translabirinthine approaches. Otherwise, a reconstruction with cartilage or fascia of the can be considered.

TRANSOTIC ENDOSCOPE-ASSISTED APPROACH

This approach allows the removal of big lesions that completely involve the petrous bone and provoke hearing loss (ie, cholesterol granulomas). In particular, endoscope introduction is indicated for the control of the paraclival region and for the control of the carotid artery at the level of the clivus and the petrous apex, allowing a good control of the petrous bone medially and anteriorly to the vertical tract of the carotid artery and to the inferior and medial tract of the horizontal part of the artery.

Microscopic Surgical Steps

An incision is made approximately 2 to 3 cm from the retroauricular groove and tissues covering the mastoid are raised. Mastoidectomy is done by the canal wall-down technique. During this phase it is important to identify the classic landmarks, such as middle cranial fossa dura, which is skeletonized posteriorly up to the sinodural angle, and the sigmoid sinus, lying posteriorly and inferiorly. Skeletonization of the sigmoid sinus proceeds in an inferior and medial direction, until the identification and skeletonization of the posterior cranial fossa dura, close to the bony labyrinth and endolymphatic sac. The sigmoid sinus is skeletonized inferiorly until a good exposition of the jugular bulb is obtained. Tympanic membrane with ossicular chain and skin of the external auditory canal is removed. The next step is the identification and skeletonization of the mastoid and tympanic tract of the facial nerve, until the geniculate ganglion is visualized above the cochleariform process, maintaining a thin bony layer to protect the nerve. Based on the extent of the pathologic condition, a drilling of the intersinus facial air cells, then a labyrinthectomy is performed, until the dura of the internal auditory canal is identified. Drilling is also extended at the retrofacial recess, creating a communication with the cochlear region and tympanic cavity. Next, a wide skeletonization of the vertical tract of the carotid artery is performed. If the lesion or pathologic matter is very extended, it is advisable to drill anteriorly to the carotid itself toward tubaric region to isolate that vessel completely. Then the stapes is removed and the vestibule is identified, the promontory is drilled until the cochlea is identified and opened. If necessary, a wide drilling of the cochlea is performed until the internal auditory canal fundus is visualized.

Endoscopic Surgical Steps

The advantage of endoscopic approach after the previous microscopic time is that it allows a precise and extended drilling at the pericartoid level, reaching anteriorly and medially to vertical tract of the carotid artery, and inferiorly to the horizontal carotid artery without extensive manipulation of the vessel itself. This procedure is indicated when the pathologic state involves the petrous apex, going toward the most medial and anterior part of the carotid artery.

Before the endoscopic procedure is started under endoscopic view, the surgical field is evaluated to obtain a good orientation. The main surgical landmarks to consider are: cochlea, vertical tract of carotid artery, tensor tympani muscle, geniculate ganglion, and jugular bulb (if it extends to the tympanic cavity) (**Fig. 3**).

Cochleariform process with tensor tympani muscle are removed to obtain a wide access to the sovratubaric region, the greater petrosal nerve is identified following the geniculate ganglion anteriorly: this latter structure is often adherent to the middle cranial fossa, which at this level becomes lower. The greater petrosal nerve is the superior limit of the dissection, representing an important landmark for internal carotid artery in its horizontal portion. The greater petrosal nerve indicates where the horizontal tract of the carotid artery can be found. When the greater petrosal nerve is followed, it can be damaged due to its fragility.

Next, drilling of the area included by vertical tract of carotid artery anteriorly, cochlea posteriorly, greater petrosal nerve superiorly, and jugular bulb inferiorly is performed.

Using 45° optics by a diamond burr the vertical tract of the carotid artery is further skeletonized, removing bone medially to the vessel. This procedure allows opening of the paraclival air cells close to the clivus. Drilling is made inferiorly and superiorly until the horizontal tract is identified, and is followed medially and anteriorly just to the anterior carotid foramen.

Drilling under endoscopic view is performed at the level of cochlear pericarotic area until a good access is obtained for instruments and optics. Drilling is continued medially to the internal carotid artery until the air cells of the petrous apex and clivus are reached. Once the air cells lying intracarotid and pericartoid have been drilled, the pathologic matter is removed by curved dissectors and suction. Neuronavigator-guided surgery can be extremely useful during these steps. Moreover, the endoscopic-assisted transotic approach 45° optic allows the best control of the retrofacial area after posterior retrofacial tympanotomy, guaranteeing the complete removal of the pathologic matter without the necessity of facial rerouting, such as happens during classic exclusively microscopic transcochlear approaches (**Fig. 3**).

Once the endoscopic procedure is ended, and after further explorative endoscopy to identify possible residuals, an obliteration of the eustachian tube is made by a temporalis muscle fragment and by obliterating the surgical cavity with abdominal fat, as

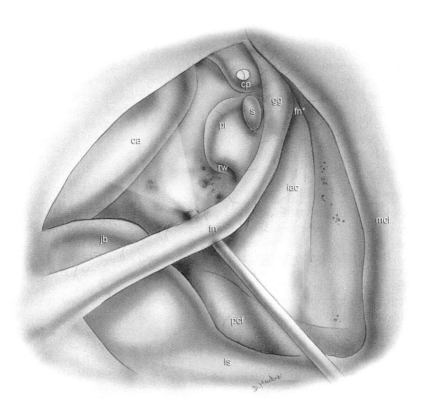

Fig. 3. (*Left ear*) The surgical cavity after transotic endoscope-assisted approach. ca, carotid artery; cp, cochleariform process; fn, facial nerve; fn*, intralabyrinthine facial nerve; gg, geniculate ganglion; iac, internal auditory canal; Jb, jugular bulb; ls, lateral sinus; lsc, lateral semicircular canal; mcf, middle cranial fossa; pcf, posterior cranial fossa; pr, promontory; rw, round window; s, stapes.

in transcochlear microscopic approaches. The procedure concludes by cul-de-sac closure of the external ear canal skin.

INFRALABYRINTHINE ENDOSCOPE-ASSISTED APPROACH

This approach is indicated for lesions extending inferiorly to the labyrinth. This approach allows removal of pathological matter without loss of hearing.

Microscopic Surgical Steps

An incision is made approximately 2 to 3 cm from the retroarticular groove and tissues covering mastoid are raised. A classic cortical mastoidectomy to underline conventional surgical landmarks, middle cranial fossa dura, and sigmoid sinus is performed. Also, the jugular bulb must be found. The mastoid tract of the facial nerve is identified anteriorly to the digastric ridge. If necessary, an antrotomy is performed and, after individuation of otic capsule and fossa incudis, the mastoidectomy is completed by removing bone more medially, toward posterior semicircular canal, which represents the superior limit of the dissection.

The purpose of these steps is to create room for the optics introduction and the following anatomic limits are eventually identified for the endoscopic dissection: superiorly the labyrinth, anteriorly and laterally the facial nerve (mastoid tract), posteriorly and inferiorly the posterior cranial fossa dura and sigmoid sinus with jugular bulb (**Fig. 4**). The next steps are endoscopic, allowing optimal pathologic tissue removal.

Endoscopic Surgical Steps

Endoscopic access is performed initially by inserting the endoscope under the retro-facial recess; bent surgical instruments (ie, dissectors) and curved suction instruments allow removal of the pathology under direct visualization by endoscopic view.

A preliminary endoscopic exploration is performed to identify landmarks. Special attention should be paid to internal auditory canal dura, which can be found at the most superior part of the field. The identification of the carotid artery is necessary in cases in which that vessel is in close relationship to the pathologic matter. Endoscopic dissection proceeds in a lateral to medial direction without damaging the labyrinth.

Initially the use of 0° optics is suggested, then 45° to explore the least accessible areas. Cleansing of the surgical filed is suggested to obtain best visualization, avoiding

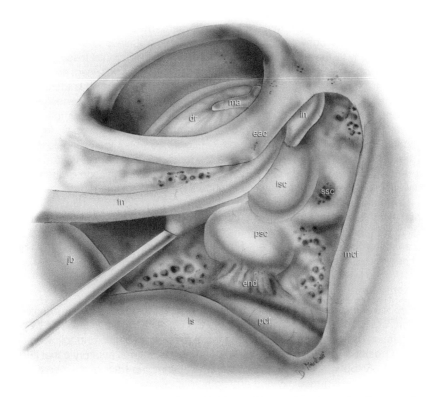

Fig. 4. (*Left ear*) The surgical cavity after infralabyrinthine endoscope-assisted approach. dr, eardrum; eac, external auditory canal; end, endolymphatic sac; fn, facial nerve; in, incus; jb, jugular bulb; ls, lateral sinus; lsc, lateral semicircular canal; ma, malleus; mcf, middle cranial fossa; pcf, posterior cranial fossa; psc, posterior semicircular canal; ssc, superior semicircular canal.

dirtying of the optic tip. Once the pathologic matter is removed, a final exploration of the surgical cavity is performed by 45° to possibly identify residuals.

At the end of the procedure, the internal ear is filled by adipose tissue and isolated from the middle ear. A middle ear obliteration by fat tissue is required only in cases of an intradural operation with extensive communication with arachnoidal spaces. This is done by eustachian tube orifice closure with muscle fragments and cul-de-sac closure of the external ear canal skin.

A contraindication to this approach can be a high jugular bulb extending superiorly and in close relationship with the labyrinth. This condition may prevent the retrofacial tympanotomy and room for endoscopic maneuvering could be reduced. Also, pathologic matter with wide intradural extension is a contraindication to this approach.

SUPRAMEATAL TRANSLABYRINTHINE ENDOSCOPE-ASSISTED APPROACH

This approach is indicated for pathologic conditions (mainly cholesteatomas) with supralabyrinthine and labyrinthine extension, with or without internal auditory canal involvement.

Microscopic Surgical Steps

An incision is made approximately 2 to 3 cm from retroarticular groove and tissues covering mastoid are raised. Mastoidectomy is performed using a canal wall down technique to identify conventional landmarks. The lateral sinus is skeletonized and followed inferiorly till the jugular bulb is identified. The middle cranial fossa is skeletonized. A good visualization of the mastoid tract of facial nerve is obtained, and the nerve is followed from mastoid tract to geniculate ganglion. The labyrinth is identified and dura of the posterior cranial fossa is skeletonized posteriorly. The endolymphatic sac is identified. The cochleariform process is removed and the tensor tympani muscle is elevated and transposed anteriorly, paying attention to not damage during procedures facial nerve. Next, a labyrinthectomy is performed until the vestibule is identified; then, the internal auditory canal dura is identified. At this level the labyrinthine tract of the facial nerve is carefully identified; the apparent direction of the nerve at this level is superiorly to inferiorly, laying superiorly to the middle turn of the cochlea until it enters into the internal auditory canal. Due to the position and orientation of the nerve at this level, the procedure is done endoscopically, identifying the geniculate ganglion with the labyrinthine tract of the facial nerve, until it enters into internal auditory canal; the close relationship between the vestibule and the labyrinthine tract of the facial nerve is also endoscopically investigated (**Fig. 5**).

Endoscopic Surgical Steps

The purpose of the endoscopic step is to remove pathologic tissue from the geniculate ganglion region and from labyrinthine tract of the facial nerve, when involved by pathologic tissue. The labyrinthine tract of the facial nerve is identified and followed anteriorly and posteriorly, lateral to medial direction, to the internal auditory canal (**Fig. 5**). The use of 45° optic allows control of the intralabyrinthine tract of the nerve and of anatomic areas laying medially and anteriorly to it, allowing matrix removal possibly without rerouting the facial nerve, which is otherwise necessary in case of a exclusive microscopic approach. This advantage includes a reduced manipulation of the nerve with a better outcome in terms of facial nerve postoperative function.

If cholesteatoma does not involve the internal auditory canal dura, the dura layer is preserved, avoiding CSF leak. On the other hand, in case of dural involvement by

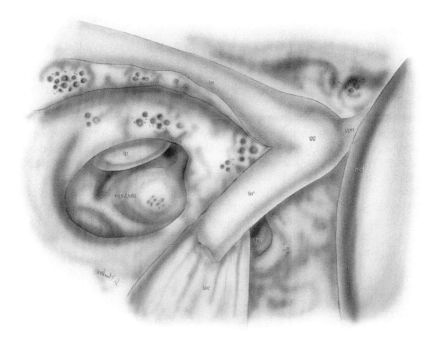

Fig. 5. (*Right ear*) The surgical cavity after suprameatal translabyrinthine endoscope-assisted approach. cho, cochlear nerve; fn, facial nerve; fn*, intralabyrinthine facial nerve; fp, stapes from behind; gg, geniculate ganglion; gpn, greater petrosal nerve; iac, internal auditory canal; mcf, middle cranial fossa.

pathologic matter, the lesion could be closed by a muscular fragment put on the surgical cavity.

The tympanic cavity and mastoid are obliterated by abdominal fat and the eustachian tube is closed by a muscle fragment. External auditory canal is closed by cul-de-sac.

SUMMARY

Use of the endoscope may benefit the surgeon in several ways for lateral skull base approaches. Its use is exclusive or in combination with microscope. Introduction of the endoscope, in the authors' opinion, can help in tissue preservation and removal of the pathologic matter, particularly in hidden areas or inaccessible spaces of the petrous bone.

REFERENCES

1. Marchioni D, Alicandri-Ciufelli M, Piccinini A, et al. Inferior retrotympanum revisited: an endoscopic anatomic study. Laryngoscope 2010;120:1880–6.
2. Tarabichi M. Endoscopic management of limited attic cholesteatoma. Laryngoscope 2004;114(7):1157–62.
3. Marchioni D, Grammatica A, Alicandri-Ciufelli M, et al. The contribution of selective dysventilation to attical middle ear pathology. Med Hypotheses 2011;77(1):116–20.

4. Marchioni D, Alicandri-Ciufelli M, Molteni G, et al. Selective epitympanic dysventilation syndrome. Laryngoscope 2010;120(5):1028–33.

5. Alicandri-Ciufelli M, Marchioni D, Grammatica A, et al. Tympanoplasty: an up-to-date pictorial review. J Neuroradiol 2012;39:149–57.

6. Marchioni D, Alicandri-Ciufelli M, Piccinini A, et al. Surgical anatomy of transcanal endoscopic approach to the tympanic facial nerve. Laryngoscope 2011;121(7): 1565–73.

7. Marchioni D, Alicandri-Ciufelli M, Molteni G, et al. Endoscopic tympanoplasty in patients with attic retraction pockets. Laryngoscope 2010;120:1847–55.

8. Marchioni D, Villari D, Alicandri-Ciufelli M, et al. Endoscopic open technique in patients with middle ear cholesteatoma. Eur Arch Otorhinolaryngol 2011; 268(11):1557–63.

9. Thomassin JM, Korchia D, Doris JM. Endoscopic guided otosurgery in the prevention of residual cholesteatomas. Laryngoscope 1993;103:939–43.

10. Presutti L, Marchioni D, Mattioli F, et al. Endoscopic management of acquired cholesteatoma: our experience. J Otolaryngol Head Neck Surg 2008;37(4): 481–7.

Endoscopic Management of Attic Cholesteatoma
A Single-Institution Experience

Daniele Marchioni, MD*, Domenico Villari, MD,
Francesco Mattioli, MD, Matteo Alicandri-Ciufelli, MD,
Alessia Piccinini, MD, Livio Presutti, MD

KEYWORDS

- Transcanal endoscopic approach • Cholesteatoma • Attic retraction
- Middle ear surgery • Residual • Recurrence

KEY POINTS

- Most spaces considered to be difficult to access with the microscopic technique could be easily visualized by endoscope-assisted surgery.
- The surgical approach should be tailored to the anatomic and physiologic concepts behind the genesis of the attic cholesteatoma, respecting as much as possible the physiology and anatomy of the middle ear.
- Middle ear folds may play an important role in the blockage of ventilation routes, possibly provoking sectorial epitympanic dysventilation.
- When isthmus blockage occurs, ventilation of the epitympanum may be impaired, and the only gas exchange would come from the mucosa of mastoid cells, excluding air provision from the Eustachian tube.

INTRODUCTION

Surgical management of cholesteatoma remains a controversial issue. Classical concepts are based on microscopic surgical management, as is the traditional classification of open tympanoplasties (canal wall down [CWD]) and closed tympanoplasties (canal wall up [CWU]), depending on the preservation of the posterior ear canal wall. The choice between these 2 techniques is based on several factors, although in most cases, the main factors influencing surgeons' ultimate attitude toward surgical management of cholesteatoma are their experience, personal beliefs, and confidence with each technique.

All the authors have read and approved the manuscript. The authors have no financial relationship to disclose.
Otolaryngology Department, University Hospital of Modena, Via del Pozzo 71, Modena 41100, Italy
* Corresponding author.
E-mail address: marchionidaniele@yahoo.it

Otolaryngol Clin N Am 46 (2013) 201–209
http://dx.doi.org/10.1016/j.otc.2012.10.004
0030-6665/13/$ – see front matter © 2013 Elsevier Inc. All rights reserved.

oto.theclinics.com

Endoscopic instrumentation, techniques, and knowledge have really improved during the past few years, and we believe that, in the future, endoscopic surgical techniques will gain increasing importance in otologic surgery. From our 7-year experience in endoscopic ear surgery, we believe that most of the spaces considered to be difficult to access with the microscopic technique could be easily visualized by endoscope-assisted surgery and we feel that new anatomic concepts should be introduced in preparation for this. From this perspective, classical concepts of CWU and CWD tympanoplasty could be completely changed in clinical practice.

When a new technique is introduced, acceptable results are essential to have it accepted by the scientific community. Because endoscopic ear surgery is a relatively "just-born" technique, only few articles reporting results are present in the literature.[1,2] This article illustrates the principles and results at our institution regarding endoscopic treatment of attic cholesteatoma.

MATERIAL AND METHODS

In January 2006, a database was created by the authors D.V. and D.M., in which all patients operated for middle ear surgery were included and followed up at our clinic by regular visits at appropriate timing (generally, after 1, 3, 6, and 12 months from the operation, then annually). At follow-up, patients were evaluated by endoscopic office examination. Noted in the database were recurrences (defined as non–self cleaning re-retraction of the attic requiring surgery) and residuals (defined as insufficient primary resection of the epidermal matrix, presenting in absence of re-retraction of the tympanic membrane). Residuals were also defined by computed tomographic evaluations, performed most frequently at 1-year follow-up. In May 2012, the database was reviewed and 321 endoscopic procedures for middle ear pathologic condition were analyzed. Of these, 253 were middle ear cholesteatomas. For the present study, only attic cholesteatomas treated endoscopically (exclusively or combined) with at least 1.5 years of follow-up were included for further analyses. Patients who had prior middle ear operations at clinical history were excluded from the analyses.

STATISTICAL ANALYSIS

Pearson correlation coefficient was used to evaluate the correlation between the absence or presence of disease (residual or recurrence) and age of patients (less than or greater than age 18 years) or type of matrix (infiltrative or sac matrix), the correlation between the absence or the residual disease and the extent of disease (cholesteatoma limited to the attic, mesotympanum extension, antral extension, mastoid extension), and the correlation between the absence or the recurrence of disease and the kind of reconstruction (cartilage, bone or fascia). The software, SPSS Statistics, version 17.0 was used for statistical analyses.

RESULTS

The final study group included 146 ears (from 146 patients). The mean follow-up was 31.2 months (DS ± 15.8). Of the 146 patients, 135 (92.5%) were free from disease at their last follow-up visit, 4 (2.7%) patients were diagnosed with recurrence, and 7 (4.8%) patients had residual disease (**Fig. 1**).

Of the 146 patients, 120 (82.2%) underwent exclusive endoscopic approach and 26 (17.8%) underwent an endoscopic approach combined with mastoidectomy (**Fig. 2**). Of 146 patients, 34 (23.3%) underwent a cholesteatoma limited exclusively to the

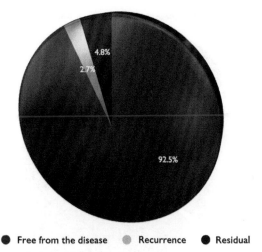

Fig. 1. Circular diagram showing the follow-up results.

attic, while 56 patients (38.4%) also had a mesotympanic extension of the disease, 32 (21.9%) had antral extension, and 24 (16.4%) had mastoid extension.

Of the 146 patients, 14 (9.6%) (**Fig. 3**) were younger than 18 years, whereas 132 (90.4%) were adults.

The cholesteatoma matrix was infiltrative in 117 of 146 patients (80.1%); 29 of 146 (19.9%) patients had a sac matrix. In 39 patients (26.7%), it was possible to avoid ossicular removal, whereas in 107 patients (73.3%), ossicular removal and reconstruction was necessary (in these cases, an ossicular chain erosion or an infiltrative matrix of the medial aspect of the ossicles was found). A total of 77 patients had a cartilage reconstruction of scutum (52.7%); in 21 patients, the reconstruction was performed by bone (14.4%) and in 48 (32.9%), by temporalis fascia (**Figs. 4–6**).

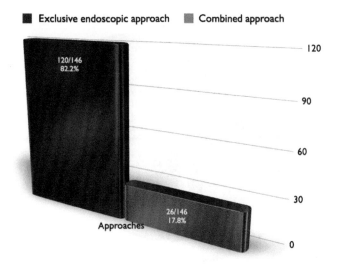

Fig. 2. Chart showing the surgical approaches.

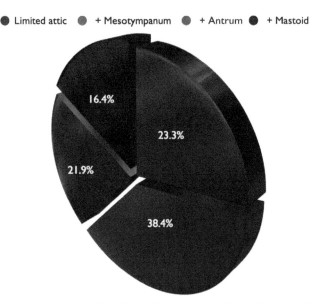

Fig. 3. Circular diagram showing the site of cholesteatoma; blue, limited to the attic; dark green, attic and mesotympanum; red, violet, attic and antrum; red, attic and mastoid.

Based on our statistical analyses, none of the variable analysis had a statistically significant impact on recurrence or residual. Regarding age (older or younger than 18 years), a recurrence or residual was present in 10 of 132 adult patients, whereas there was 1 case of recurrence of 14 patients aged younger than 18 years ($P = .95$). Regarding the type of matrix, out of 28 patients with sac matrix, none experienced residual or recurrence, whereas 7 of 114 patients with infiltrative matrix experienced residual or recurrence ($P = .17$). Of 33 patients with cholesteatoma limited exclusively to the attic, none experienced residual, and of 55 patients who also had

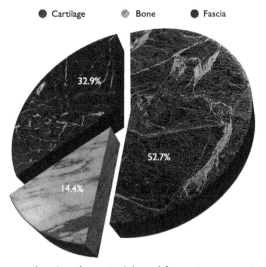

Fig. 4. Circular diagram showing the material used for scutum reconstruction.

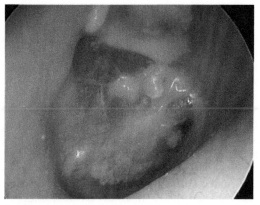

Fig. 5. Twenty-month follow-up of an exclusive endoscopic approach with cartilage scutum reconstruction.

a mesotympanic extension, 2 experienced residual pathologic condition at follow-up. Of 31 patients with antral extension, 2 experienced residual, and of 23 patients with mastoid extension, 3 experienced residual (overall *P* value considering subsite extension = 0.15). Of 75 patients who had a cartilage reconstruction of the scutum, 2 experienced recurrence; of 19 patients who had a bone reconstruction of the scutum, 1 experienced recurrence. Of 45 patients who had temporalis facia reconstruction, 1 experienced recurrence (overall *P* value considering reconstruction = 0.79).

DISCUSSION

Primary acquired cholesteatoma is usually a manifestation of advanced retraction of the tympanic membrane that occurs when the sac advances into the tympanic cavity proper and then into its extensions such as the sinus tympani, the facial recess, the hypotympanum, and the attic.[3]

Only in advanced cases does a cholesteatoma progress further to reach the mastoid cavity. Most surgical failures associated with a postauricular approach seem to occur within the tympanic cavity, and it is difficult to reach that extension rather than the localization at the mastoid region.

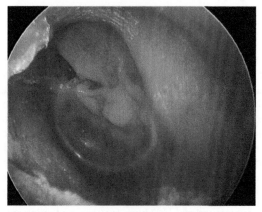

Fig. 6. Twelve-month follow-up of a combined approach with cartilage scutum reconstruction.

The main problems regarding attic cholesteatoma removal are residual and recurrence.

Residual is due to insufficient primary resection of the epidermal matrix and classically presents a pearl-like appearance. Insufficient resection may be the result of a very fine epidermal matrix, middle ear inflammation, and particularly, a limited exposition of hidden areas such as epitympanic space and sinus tympani. The view during microscopic surgery is defined and limited by the narrowest segment of the ear canal; this basic limitation has forced surgeons to create a parallel port through the mastoid to gain keyhole access to the attic. Despite the illumination and magnification offered by the operating microscope, it has proved to have distinct limitations.

The surgeon can visualize structures only directly ahead and is unable to see "around-the-corner" objects. So this straight-line view offered by the microscope result in certain blind pockets during middle ear surgery. These limitations can be overcome with the complementary help of an endoscope.[4] Thomassin and colleagues[5] found that by using intraoperative endoscopy, the quality of disease eradication significantly improved and resulted in the decrease in incidence of residual cholesteatoma from 47% to 6%. Youssef and Poe[6] found that the use of the endoscopic technique significantly decreased the morbidity of the second-look procedure, enhanced visualization of residual disease, and reduced operating time. Badr-El-Dine[7] reported on the value of endoscopy as an adjunct in cholesteatoma surgery and documented a reduced risk of residuals when the endoscope was used. In the primary surgery, after completion of microscopic cleaning, the overall incidence of intraoperative residuals detected with the endoscope was 22.8%; sinus tympani was the most common site of intraoperative residuals in both CWU and CWD groups. At second-look endoscopic explorations, 8.6% of recurrences were identified.

The recurrence consists in a new dangerous tympanic retraction pocket caused by inadequate reconstruction of scutum and tympanic loss of substance, inducing persistence of the physiopathologic process of middle ear depression.

Recurrence can be diagnosed otoscopically, whereas residual cholesteatoma is classically independent of the eardrum and only surgical revision can determine definite diagnosis; this is the rationale of the second-look procedures, beside functional issues.[8] The persistence of physiopathologic phenomena, which had determined the cholesteatoma development, presents as a new attic retraction, which requires a further surgical approach to avoid the re-formation of attic cholesteatoma.

Cholesteatoma surgery primarily aims to eradicate the disease process and provide the patient with a safe and dry ear.

In cholesteatoma surgery, 2 competitive techniques have developed over the course of time:

1. Closed "CWU" tympanoplasty preserves physiologic epidermis migration from the inner portion of the external auditory canal and prevents infectious complications resulting from an unstable drainage cavity. These features make it the technique of choice in middle ear cholesteatoma. It entails, however, a risk of residual cholesteatoma ranging from 10% to 40%,[9–13] requiring radiological surveillance and/or second-look surgery, and this technique is not without recurrence rate.
2. Open "CWD" tympanoplasty allows excellent visualization of the disease with a proportionally good chance of complete removal but not without a residual rate, and it has a much less frequent recurrence rate. The disadvantage of the procedure is the lifelong need for frequent cleaning of the open cavity and water restrictions.

In the literature, several works[5,7,14,15] have focused on the intraoperative use of the endoscope during traditional microscopic CWU and CWD.

The endoscope-assisted surgery allows the surgeon to opt for a more conservative CWU, instead of CWD. Moreover, considering also that a CWD does not always allow exploration of hidden areas, the systematic intraoperative use of the endoscope is also useful in CWD mastoidectomy.[15]

Despite the anatomic and physiologic function of the connection between mastoid and middle ear, in both these surgical procedures, the surgeon needs to remove the mastoid cells and mucosa to reach the cholesteatoma from behind. From our 7-year experience in endoscopic ear surgery, we feel that new anatomic concepts should be introduced for better treating the pathologic condition of the ear. In this perspective, classical concepts of CWU and CWD tympanoplasties could be completely changed on clinical practice.

Despite the tools of choice, to be used during the surgery of the middle ear cholesteatoma, the surgical approach should be tailored to the anatomic and physiologic concepts that generate attic cholesteatoma, preserving as much as possible the physiology and the anatomy of the middle ear. These concepts may be crucial to get an optimal "functional result."

From our previous experiences,[14,16] the key in attic cholesteatoma is the correct comprehension of physiopathologic pathways. Epitympanum aeration is strictly dependent on the ventilation pathways clarified by Palva and Ramsay,[17] and possible selective dysventilation of epitympanic compartments could provoke attic retractions or cholesteatoma.

When an isthmus blockage occurs, ventilation of the epitympanum may be impaired, and the only gas exchange would come from the mucosa of mastoid cells, excluding air provision from the Eustachian tube. We recently studied middle ear ventilation route blockage and its relationship with mastoid pneumatization, and some different types of isthmus blockage, related to different pathologic conditions, were identified and classified.[18] Moreover, we found that obstruction of the tympanic isthmus is a consistent finding in patients affected by limited attic cholesteatoma.

In the past years, several studies have focused on evaluating the role of tympanic isthmus, especially in cadaveric dissection studies[14,18]; with the advent of endoscopic techniques, it has become possible to study the morphologic shape of the epitympanic diaphragm and tympanic isthmus in the pathologic ears especially in case of attic cholesteatoma. This would have been impossible by a microscope because of the angulation and the position of tympanic isthmus. From these studies, it was clear how, in patients with epitympanic cholesteatoma, a complete epitympanic diaphragm was present, associated to a total isthmus blockage, and this created a complete ventilatory exclusion of the epitympanic compartments from the mesotympanic spaces, causing a low ossigenation of the mucosa of the attic space and mastoid compartments, which is in general guaranteed by the Eustachian tube. The low ventilation would generate a progressive air reabsorbtion through the attic mucosa, creating a selective epitympanic negative pressure in the attic that could be the pathogenetic substrate for the complete pars flaccida retraction to the lateral attic space and the progressive formation of attic cholesteatoma. This could explain the typical clinical scenario of an attic cholesteatoma or attic retraction associated with the erosion of the scutum, with a normal shape and position of the pars tensa and without pathologic alteration in mesotympanum. Actually, middle ear folds may play an important role in the blockage of ventilation routes, possibly provoking sectorial epitympanic dysventilation.[14,18] So systematic intraoperative visualization, analysis, and in some cases, removal of these folds, should be mandatory in every procedure. Preservation of mastoid tissue may contribute to improvement of postoperative middle ear ventilation, because of their role in middle ear gas exchange. From these concepts, we believe that the surgical approach to attic cholesteatoma should respect some conditions: disease eradication with direct access to the hidden areas, preservation of the mastoid cells and mucosa wherever possible, and restoration of the physiologic aeration pathways from the Eustachian tube to the attic, by removing the block of the isthmus and by creating additional aeration pathways through the tensor fold (which connects the protympanum to the anterior attic). From all these concepts, we strongly believe that we need to develop a direct surgical approach through the external auditory canal to the middle ear cholesteatoma, and the endoscope at present is the best tool to allow a direct access to the tympanic cavity areas, getting also a direct view of the isthmus and tensor fold areas. When cholesteatoma is limited to the tympanic cavity, the transcanal endoscopic approach allows the eradication of the disease, the ventilation routes being restored by removing the isthmus blockage and the tensor fold, while preserving the mastoid mucosa.

Exclusive endoscopic tympanoplasty was first described by Tarabichi.[19] The new concept of endoscopic ear surgery redirected the attention away from the less-critical areas (ie, mastoid) toward the tympanic cavity and its "hard-to-reach" extensions. The endoscopic technique was codified for a minimally invasive eradication of limited attic cholesteatoma, preserving the ossicular chain wherever possible with complete removal of the disease. From this indication, the clinical application of the transcanal endoscopic approach has allowed to extend the indication of this technique to cholesteatoma of the whole tympanic cavity without mastoid involvement.

Some disadvantages of endoscopic technique must be considered:

- The endoscopic approach is a "one-hand technique"; for this reason, surgeons need special learning curve to improve their personal skills.
- The mastoid is not accessible by the endoscope, and when the mastoid is involved with the cholesteatoma, a microscopic technique is required.

Regarding our results, none of the comparisons (matrix, age, subsite involvement, type of reconstruction) considered until now have reached a statistically significant value. The authors would attribute this finding more to the small sample size or to the rarity of the events (recurrence or residual) than to the real absence of differences between factors considered. The authors would like to underline that further experiences and longer follow-up are for sure necessary to confirm and underline factors possibly influencing results. Regarding recurrence rates and residual pathologic conditions, the "middle-term results" of our cohort of patients are completely similar to those reported in the literature for microscopic surgery of cholesteatoma, especially regarding the recurrence rate.

The authors are convinced that the main issue is the preservation of the graft used to reconstruct the scutum. Understanding the behavior and healing process of the graft during the follow-up time is crucial, to understand if the preservation of the buffer mastoid mechanism and the restoration of attic ventilation are useful to maintain the graft in the original position without developing recurrent attic retraction.

SUMMARY

Endoscopic ear surgery can be considered an effective method to eradicate cholesteatoma from middle ear. It guarantees better visualization of hidden areas, better chances of tissue preservation, and minimally invasive access. It also allows better understanding of the pathophysiology of cholesteatoma, along with a detailed anatomic study. Results are comparable to those reported for microscopic techniques in terms of recurrences or residual pathology. Further experiences are necessary to confirm our results.

REFERENCES

1. Migirov L, Shapira Y, Horowitz Z, et al. Exclusive endoscopic ear surgery for acquired cholesteatoma: preliminary results. Otol Neurotol 2011;32(3):433–6.
2. Tarabichi M. Endoscopic management of cholesteatoma: long-term results. Otolaryngol Head Neck Surg 2000;122(6):874–81.
3. Sheehy JL, Brackmann DE, Graham MD. Cholesteatoma surgery: residual and recurrent disease. A review of 1,024 cases. Ann Otol Rhinol Laryngol 1977;86: 451–62.
4. Magnan J, Chays A, Lepetre C, et al. Surgical perspectives of endoscopy of the cerebellopontine angle. Am J Otol 1994;15:366–70.
5. Thomassin JM, Korchia D, Doris JM. Endoscopic-guided otosurgery in the prevention of residual cholesteatomas. Laryngoscope 1993;103:939–43.
6. Youssef TF, Poe DS. Endoscope-assisted second-stage tympanomastoidectomy. Laryngoscope 1997;107:1341–4.
7. Badr-el-Dine M. Value of ear endoscopy in cholesteatoma surgery. Otol Neurotol 2002;23:631–5.
8. Gaillardin L, Lescanne E, Morinière S, et al. Residual cholesteatoma: prevalence and location. Follow-up strategy in adults. Eur Ann Otorhinolaryngol Head Neck Dis 2012;129(3):136–40.
9. Haginomori S, Takamaki A, Nonaka R, et al. Residual cholesteatoma: incidence and localization in canal wall down tympanoplasty with soft-wall reconstruction. Arch Otolaryngol Head Neck Surg 2008;134:652–7.
10. Barakate M, Bottrill I. Combined approach tympanoplasty for cholesteatoma: impact of middle ear endoscopy. J Laryngol Otol 2008;122:120–4.
11. Hinohira Y, Yanahigara N, Gyo K. Improvements to staged canal wall up tympanoplasty for middle ear cholesteatoma. Otolaryngol Head Neck Surg 2007;137: 913–7.
12. Hamilton JW. Efficacy of the KTP laser in the treatment of middle ear cholesteatoma. Otol Neurotol 2005;26:135–9.
13. Yung MW. The use of middle ear endoscopy: has residual cholesteatoma been eliminated? J Laryngol Otol 2001;115:958–61.
14. Marchioni D, Mattioli F, Alicandri Ciufelli M, et al. Endoscopic approach to tensor fold in patients with attic cholesteatoma. Acta Otolaryngol 2009;129:946–54.
15. Presutti L, Marchioni D, Mattioli F, et al. Endoscopic management of acquired cholesteatoma: our experience. J Otolaryngol Head Neck Surg 2008;37(4): 481–7.
16. Marchioni D, Alicandri Ciufelli M, Molteni G, et al. Selective epitympanic dysventilation syndrome. Laryngoscope 2010;120:1028–33.
17. Palva T, Ramsay H. Chronic inflammatory ear disease and cholesteatoma: creation of auxiliary attic aeration pathways by microdissection. Am J Otol 1999;20: 145–51.
18. Marchioni D, Mattioli F, Alicandri-Ciufelli M, et al. Endoscopic evaluation of middle ear ventilation route blockage. Am J Otolaryngol 2010;31(6):453–66.
19. Tarabichi M. Endoscopic management of acquired cholesteatoma. Am J Otol 1997;18:5444–9.

Instrumentation and Technologies in Endoscopic Ear Surgery

Mohamed Badr-El-Dine, MD[a],*,
Adrian L. James, MA, DM, FRCS(ORL-HNS)[b], Giuseppe Panetti, MD[c,d],
Daniele Marchioni, MD[c], Livio Presutti, MD[c], João Flávio Nogueira[e]

KEYWORDS

- Endoscopic ear surgery • Microscopic ear surgery • Otologic instruments
- Cholesteatoma

KEY POINTS

- The operating microscope requires wide viewing portals for adequate illumination and visualization of the operative field, contrary to the endoscope, which provides direct vision with illumination to the target field, thus avoiding the need for extra exposure and extra drilling.
- When planning an exclusive endoscopic ear surgery, still the microscope is an essential part of the surgical setting making it ready to use whenever needed. Combining the attributes of microscope and endoscope during surgery is the most efficacious approach.
- Cholesteatoma resection is considered complete only after a final survey with the angled endoscopes is completed, confirming absence of pathologic conditions from all hidden recesses.
- The principal advantage of aspiration instruments is the ability to perform dissection and aspiration maneuvers at the same time overcoming the impact of operating with one hand as imposed by otoendoscopic surgery. The main limit of instruments with suction channels is the possibility of occlusion caused by detritus aspirated during dissection.

 Videos demonstrating use of the instrumentation discussed in this article are available at http://www.oto.theclinics.com/

INTRODUCTION

This article covers state-of-the-art devices and instruments specially designated for endoscopic ear surgery. New technologies have stimulated the creation of special endoscopic equipment and microinstruments specially designed to satisfy the

All authors have no financial associations with industry or other conflict of interest.
[a] Faculty of Medicine, University of Alexandria, 36 Rouschdy Street #6, Rouschdy, Alexandria, Egypt; [b] Department of Otolaryngology—Head and Neck Surgery, Hospital for Sick Children, University of Toronto, 555 University Avenue, Toronto, Ontario M5G 1X8, Canada; [c] Otolaryngology Department, ASCALESI Hospital, via E. a Forcella 31, Naples 80139, Italy; [d] Faculty of Medicine "Federico II" Naples, via del Parco Grifeo 40, Naples 80121, Italy; [e] Hospital Geral de Fortaleza, Brazil
* Corresponding author.
E-mail address: mbeldine@yahoo.com

Otolaryngol Clin N Am 46 (2013) 211–225
http://dx.doi.org/10.1016/j.otc.2012.10.005
0030-6665/13/$ – see front matter © 2013 Elsevier Inc. All rights reserved.

oto.theclinics.com

exclusive requirements of endoscopic ear surgery, which in turn contributes to the progress of the specialty. In addition, these new, specially designed instruments have expanded the indications and refined the surgical skills for this surgery. This, in turn, allows better control of pathological conditions and permits access to previously unreachable or difficult to reach anatomic recesses (ie, sinus tympani, facial recess, and anterior epitympanic recess).

The operating room for ear surgery should contain state-of-the-art instrumentation. The surgeon should be in a comfortable working position during the prolonged holding of the endoscope, which is mounted with the endoscopic video camera. Even when planning an exclusive endoscopic ear surgery, the microscope is an essential part of the surgical setting. The microscope should be supplied with a built-in high-definition camera that allows continuous documentation in parallel with the endoscopic surgery performed, all through a high-definition video monitor. The presence of continuous video monitoring enables the anesthesiologist, the scrub nurse, and others to observe and follow the proceedings of the operation. Recordings can also be used for teaching purposes.

The patient is placed supine on the operating room table in the normal otologic position. The microscope is placed in the sterile field ready to be used whenever needed. The endoscopic tower is placed directly facing the surgeon while the monitor is level with the surgeon's eyes. Because the surgeon is not looking down into the eyepiece of the endoscope and, instead, is looking directly forward at the video screen, proper alignment of these components is essential to keep the surgeon orientated to the surgical field and to ensure a comfortable working position.

STANDARD INSTRUMENTS FOR MICROSCOPIC EAR SURGERY

Besides the standard instruments required for the approach through the soft tissue (eg, scalpels, forceps, and monopolar and bipolar diathermy), specific otologic instruments (**Fig. 1**) include

- Self-retaining mastoid retractors

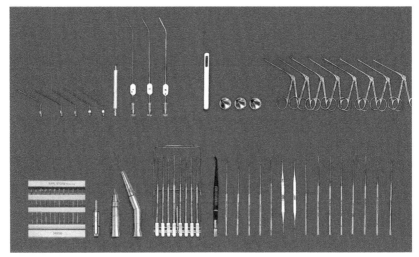

Fig. 1. Standard otologic instruments set used by otologists in all regular microscopic ear surgery. (*Courtesy of* Plester, Karl Storz GMBH & Co, Tuttlingen, Germany; with permission.)

- Instruments for bone work: microdrill, micromotor handles straight and curved, set of different-sized tungsten cutting burrs, and diamond burrs
- Irrigation and suction instruments
- Soft tissue dissectors, large and small scissors, toothed and untoothed forceps, periosteal raspatory.

In general, a full set of microsurgical instruments is required, which are very familiar to practicing otologists:

- Microforceps (microcup and microalligator); microscissors, delicate straight and curved; microhooks of different angles and lengths; needles; elevators, knives of different sizes and shapes (eg, round cutting knife); Plester vertical cutting knife; sickle knives of variable curvatures; Rosen elevator; House curettes, large and small; and so forth
- Suckers and suction-irrigation of different sizes
- Fine suction tips and adaptors with control hole.

ENDOSCOPES AND SPECIAL INSTRUMENTS FOR ENDOSCOPIC EAR SURGERY
Ear Endoscopes

Endoscopes have proved increasing benefit in ear surgery. Incorporating the endoscope into the surgical armamentarium in otology has contributed much to the concept of minimally invasive surgery. This is because the operating microscope requires wide viewing portals for adequate illumination and visualization of the operative field, contrary to endoscope, which provides direct vision with illumination to the target field, thus avoiding the need for extra exposure and extra drilling.

Endoscopes have many proven advantages over the microscope, including

- Wider angle of view
- Better visualization of structures that are parallel to the axis of the microscope
- Visualization of deep recesses and hidden structures (ie, around the corner)
- Ability to visualize beyond the shaft of the surgical instruments.

On the other hand, several disadvantages of endoscopes include[1–3]

- Loss of depth perception and binocular vision
- The inevitable one-handed surgical technique involved
- Need for a strictly bloodless field (meticulous attention to hemostasis is essential)
- Fogging and smearing of the tip of the endoscope
- The mandatory need for reliable physician training
- The cost of equipment.

Rigid Endoscopes

The design of the Hopkins rod-lens system was developed to yield endoscopes of variable length, diameters, and angles of view. The rigid endoscopes commonly used for ear surgery are 2.7 mm, 3 mm, or 4 mm in diameter. All the new endoscopes are now autoclavable. The working lengths are 18 cm, 11 cm, and 6 cm. The larger the diameter, the better the image displays and the more light it can transmit to the operative field. The 0° and 30° angled scopes are the most commonly used, followed by the 45°. Endoscopes with a greater angle, such as the 70°, are difficult and disorienting to work with and are only used for inspection in limited spots, such as the sinus tympani, which may lie very deep in 20% of cases (**Fig. 2**). Recently, new developments in optics have led to the creation of a new generation of wide-angled endoscopes with smaller diameters that provide better quality images.

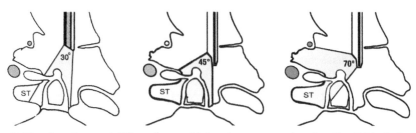

Fig. 2. The sinus tympani (ST) and pyramidal eminence area showing the field of view of different angled endoscopes and the degree of visualization each endoscope can provide.

The 0° endoscope provides all of the imaging needed to perform the major steps of any endoscopic operation. The optics allow near-complete exposure of most of the field and pathologic condition. However, the extent of visualization under the 0° endoscope is limited by its optical capabilities. The distal lens of the otoscopes must be cleaned with an antifog solution before each application.

Practically, in cholesteatoma surgery, once cholesteatoma resection under the 0° endoscope is deemed complete, it is replaced with the angled 30° or 45° endoscopes. By advancing the angled endoscope and rotating it in clockwise and counterclockwise directions along its longitudinal axis, all middle ear recesses are visualized and any hidden pathologic conditions can be detected and removed. Cholesteatoma resection is considered complete only after a final survey with the angled endoscopes is completed, confirming absence of pathologic condition. A 70° endoscope may also be used in this examination; however, in most cases, the information obtained by the 30° or 45° lens is sufficient to identify any residual pathologic condition.[4–7]

Instruments

The development of special equipment and instruments for endoscopic ear surgery is based on the International Working Group on Endoscopic Ear Surgery (IWGEES) experience of more than 15 years performing endoscope-assisted and/or exclusive endoscopic ear surgery. Adapting and refining regular microinstruments to include longer, more slender shafts with single or double curvatures and smaller microtips have been essential for endoscopic ear surgery.

Major innovation of highly sophisticated technologies such as xenon light sources, high-resolution cameras and monitors, digital processors, documentation, and lens irrigation systems have complemented the advances in endoscopic technology and stimulated the creation of dedicated endoscopic equipment and microinstruments specially designed to fulfill the unique requirements of endoscopic ear surgery.

Practically, endoscope-assisted and fully endoscopic ear surgery require the standard otologic microinstruments, familiar and used by any otologist, and the specially modified and newly designed endoscopic ear surgery instruments. A basic set of instruments, based on the IWGEES experience, used exclusively for endoscopic ear surgery is now available.[2] It includes sets of curved shaft dissectors and sharp hooks, sets of curved suction cannulae, sets of curved curettes, and sets of curved cupped forceps with 10 cm working length. Most recent are the newly designed instruments incorporating suction into the shaft, facilitating dissection with one hand while the other hand holds the endoscope. The best example of this is the round cutting knife with suction shaft (**Fig. 3**).

Classic microscopic ear surgery instruments are usually straight shaft or mild curve shaft but, because endoscopic ear surgery necessitates working with the angled

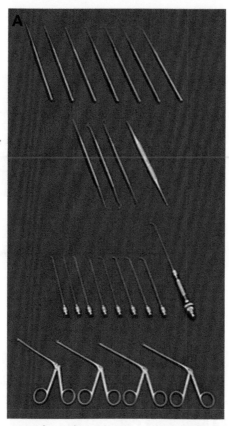

Fig. 3. (*A*) New instrument set for endoscopic ear surgery according to the IWGEES. (*B*) Newly invented suction cannulae, straight, with angled tips of different angulations and lengths. They have diameters ranging from 0.8 mm to 1.6 mm and a length of 10 cm. All are Luer-Lok to be mounted on the Fisch adaptor or the turning adaptor. A rotating adaptor is essential for easy manipulation of cannulae with angled tips. The choice of diameter for these reusable cannulae provides extra comfort for surgeon to choose the optimum instrument for the task. (*C*) Incorporating suction into the shaft of endoscopic microinstruments is a major modification that will help the single-handed surgeon overcome bleeding while dissecting or manipulating tissues and holding the endoscope with the other hand. The round cutting knife, diameter 3 mm, with suction shaft is easy to handle due to rotatable tubing connector, length 19 cm. (*D*) Set of four endoscopic fine-cupped forceps, working length 10 cm, strongly curved. Directions: right, left, backward 90°, and upward 45°. (*E*) Set of fine sharp hooks and elevators, 90°, all with strongly curved shaft and of different directions: right, left, and backward. The presence of the curve on the shaft of the instrument mandates the need for different directions; therefore, the newly designed endoscopic instruments handles are marked to allow easy identification of the direction of each instrument: one marking for right, two markings for left, and three markings for backward. These marks on the handle avoid confusion and facilitate handling of the correct instrument. (*F*) Ear hooks, sharp, 90° right, left, and backward with strongly curved shaft. (*G*) Newly designed endoscopic instruments: Elevators 90° right, left, and backward with strongly curved shaft (*left*). The presence of the curve on the shaft of the instrument mandates the need for different directions. These elevators enable atraumatic dissection of the cholesteatoma matrix from over vital middle ear structures (*right*). (*H*) Set of ear curettes of different sizes with bent shaft to facilitate working under angled vision endoscope. Single-ended curette with curved shaft, double-ended curette with 90° curved shaft, and the standard House double-ended curette. Double-ended 90° curved shaft cleaning the anterior epitympanic recess endoscope is placed transcanal (*lower left*). Double-ended 90° curved shaft cleaning the under surface of the scutum transmastoid (*lower center*). Single-ended curved curette cleaning the under surface of the scutum transcanal (*lower right*). ([A] *Courtesy of* Karl Storz GMBH & Co. KG, Mittelstraße 8, D-78532 Tuttlingen, Germany; with permission.)

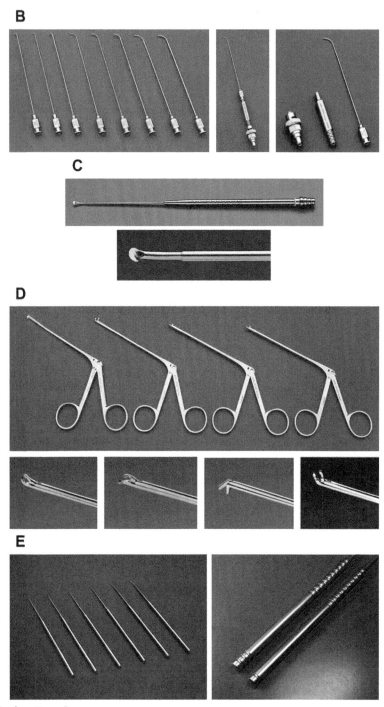

Fig. 3. (*continued*)

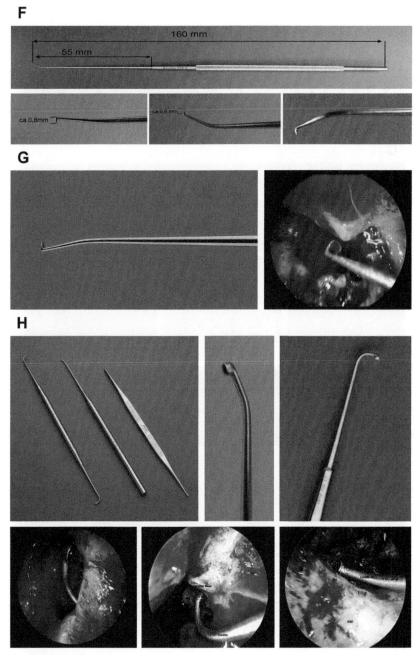

Fig. 3. (*continued*)

30° or 45° scopes (see **Fig. 2**), instruments should be fashioned accordingly with a single-bend or double-bend shaft or significantly curved shaft. This allows ease in reaching into the hidden recesses of the middle ear without the need for extra drilling merely for the sake visualization and instrument handling.

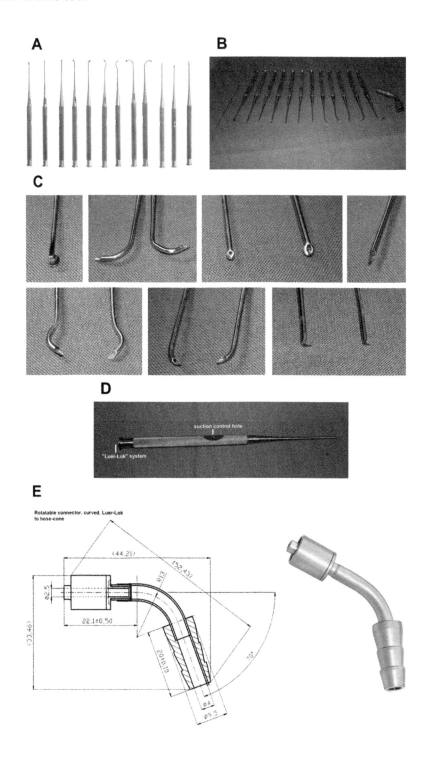

Because of the growing indications for exclusive endoscopic surgery, and because major steps are performed under angled endoscopic control, the need to modify more instruments to adapt for the angled vision endoscopic surgery (30° and 45°) proves essential.[8] The IWGEES has worked extensively to create highly specialized instrument sets specially designed for endoscopic ear surgery. More instruments specially adapted for endoscopic ear surgery are now developed. Miniaturization of some of the already existing endoscopic sinus surgery instruments is in progress to adapt for endoscopic ear surgery. Adding curvature to the shaft of microinstruments proves essential to allow the instrument to reach into the deep hidden recesses and make it possible to remove pathologic conditions "around the corner." Once the instruments acquire curved shafts, the instruments require working direction (ie, right, left, and backward). To facilitate handling of instruments of different directions, handles are marked according to the direction of the instrument tip. For instance, there is one mark for right-sided, two marks for left-sided, and three marks for backward tipped (see **Fig. 3**E). Curved forceps with 10 cm working length are also provided to improve surgical maneuverability.

Finally, incorporating suction into the instrument shaft is considered one of the most important modifications that enable the single-handed surgeon to work in a clean blood-less field. Different modifications were provided by different companies (eg, the round cutting knife with suction shaft; see **Fig. 3**C). Many other attempts were introduced to overcome the limits of single-handed endoscopic surgery. Most impressive was the instrument set developed by Professor Giuseppe Panetti in which he imagined a surgical instrument (**Fig. 4**A–D) that has the same shape and length as the traditional one but features a suction channel. Each instrument can be divided in three components:

1. Operative distal extremity
2. Handle with suction control hole
3. Proximal extremity provided with Luer-Lok connection.

The main limitation of this instrument is the possibility of occlusion caused by detritus aspirated during dissection. At the same time, the facility of instrument exchange minimizes the impact of this inconvenience.

The principal advantage of aspiration instruments is the chance to perform dissection and aspiration maneuvers at the same time. This reduces the impact of operating with one hand as imposed by otoendoscopic approach. Dissection operations turn out to be more efficient as a result of the aspiration capability of the instrument. Blurring, as well as blood spots occurring on the endoscope's extremity, which are the most

Fig. 4. (*A, B*) The Giuseppe Panetti instrument set characterized by the same shape and length as the traditional set but featuring a suction channel. (*C*) Each instrument presents a different "operative distal extremity," which recalls the most common dissection instruments shapes for the middle ear (eg, a pair of dissectors for tympanic sinus, lenticular bistoury, two lengths curved hook, 45° angled needle). Each extremity is provided with suction opening. (*D*) The intermediate portion in each instrument consists of a handle with a suction control hole. This allows a regulation of instruments aspiration capability. Proximal extremity is provided with a Luer-Lok connector that permits a rapid change of instruments depending on surgeon's needs and in case it gets occluded during dissecting maneuvers. (*E*) The connector is curved, 5 cm, 70° angled and is provided with a rotating distal extremity with a complementary Luer-Lok system. This meets specific ergonomic requirements, ensuring the maximum reduction of attrition to the weight of aspiration tube where joint's proximal extremity is hooked. This makes the instrument handle particularly comfortable and makes dissecting maneuvers easier.

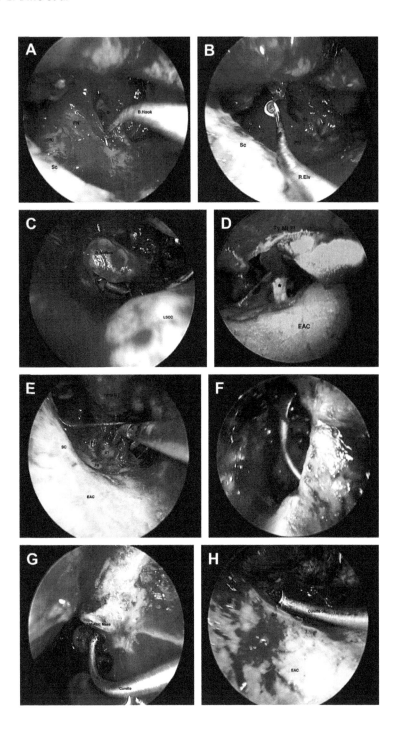

common inconveniences, can be easily removed through physiologic solution washes, assuring a constantly clean operative field without losing fluidity of surgical gestures.

The similarity between the newly designed endoscopic suction instruments and the classical otological instruments make it possible for all otology surgeons to work with ease, thus contributing to wider usage of the endoscopic procedure.

To illustrate the use of new instruments during endoscopic ear surgery, multiple endoscopic views are presented in **Fig. 5**). Videos are also presented that illustrate the technical use of these specially designed endoscopic ear instruments (Videos 1–6).

ADVANCED TECHNOLOGIES USED IN OTOLOGY SURGERY

The following advanced technologies have improved otology surgery:

1. High-definition digital cameras attached to the telescope project images onto one or several monitors. The three-chip cameras and, recently, the high-definition, fully digital cameras produce excellent quality images and feature automatic controls for color, exposure, white balance, and digital contrast enhancement. The Image 1 supplied by Karl Storz instantly converts optical images to digital with improved imaging on all digital recording and display devices. It offers the resolution and light sensitivity necessary for the highest digital image quality. The illumination is generated by a powerful cold-light source and transmitted to the endoscope via a fiber-optic light cable of 180 cm length. The different types of light sources (halogen, xenon, LED) offer light of varying brightness. Xenon is currently preferred.

◄───

Fig. 5. Endoscopic ear surgery. (*A*) Right ear view using 30° endoscope. Backward sharp hook (B. Hook) cutting adhesions between the stapes (St) and the facial nerve (FN). Notice the stapes (St), the promontory (P) and the scutum (Sc). As for the asterisk please add it in the context of the phrase: Right ear view using 30° endoscope, Right elevator (R.Elv) dissecting granulation (*) and cholesteatoma from over the facial nerve (FN) (*B*) Right ear view using 30° endoscope. Right elevator (R. Elv.) dissecting granulation and cholesteatoma from over the facial nerve (FN) and cochleariform process. Notice the lateral semicircular canal (LSSC), the stapes (St), and the scutum (Sc). (*C*) Right ear showing transmastoid endoscopic view using 30° scope, 3 mm diameter. The anterior epitympanic recess with the head of malleus attached medially by the tensor tympanic tendon is perfectly visualized. The curved suction (Crv. Suct.) cannula passing transcanal, cleaning the orifice of the eustachian tube (*asterisk*), is seen through the opening created after disrupting the tensor tympani fold. Edge of the tensor tympani fold (*double asterisk*). ant Ep Rc, anterior epitympanic recess; LSSC, lateral semicircular canal. (*D*) Left posterosuperior retraction pocket cholesteatoma. The round cutting knife with suction shaft used to dissect the tympanomeatal flap (Ty Mt Fl) is seen retracting the meatal skin and entering the middle ear. Whitish cholesteatoma matrix is seen in the retrotympanum (*asterisk*). Pm, Promontory. (*E*) Right ear view using 30° endoscope. Left-curved fine cupped forceps with 10 cm working length removing granulation tissue from over the sinus tympani (ST). Stapes head (ST H) attached by the stapedius tendon. EAC, external auditory canal; FR, facial recess; SC, scutum; Tymp MF, tympanomeatal flap. (*F*) Left ear view using 30° endoscope. Double-ended, strongly curved curette is used to clean the anterior epitympanic recess. Notice the double-approach surgery as the endoscope is placed transcanal while the curette is passing transmastoid. EAC, external auditory canal; FR, facial recess; Sc, scutum. (*G*) Right ear showing transmastoid endoscopic view using 30° scope, 3 mm diameter. Double-ended curette, 90° curved shaft while cleaning the under surface of the lateral attic mass (Lat. Attic Mass). The strongly curved curette allows the surgeon to remove pathologic conditions in deep, difficult to reach spots. Mal, head of malleus. (*H*) Right ear view using 30° endoscope. Single-ended, strong curved shaft curette (Curette SE) used to clean the undersurface of the scutum (Sc). EAC, external auditory canal; Tymp MF, tympanomeatal flap.

2. High-definition digital monitors, data management, and documentation are now considered standard equipment whenever endoscopic ear surgery is performed. The digital documentation system, Advanced Image and Data Archiving HD (AIDA), provides convenient image, video, and audio archiving of important stages and results of a procedure for patient and scientific documentation.

3. Microdrill handpieces, attachments, and burrs are used to perform different functions during middle ear surgery in combination with different sizes curettes. For endoscopic ear surgery, the pen-style, compact, powerful, lightweight, high-performance microdrills provide the balance and maneuverability that enable the surgeon to work in tight spaces. Also, the microdrill attachments are tapered to provide improved visibility of the cutting or diamond burrs at its tip during surgery.

4. Piezosurgery, specially designed for bone dissection, is manufactured by Mectron.[9] Piezosurgery, though it does not replace the micromotors for bone drilling, offers the state of the art in bone surgery. The piezoelectric ceramic disks contained in the Piezosurgery Medical handle transmit the microvibration to special inserts designed for each surgical technique. It has the advantage of minimal damage to the soft tissue, maximum surgical precision, blood-free surgical site, and maximum intraoperative visibility. The very fine movement of the cutting inserts (micrometers) enables maximum intraoperative control. It allows bone cut with only 0.3 to 0.6 mm width with no bone necrosis. The wide range of surgical inserts makes it easy to use in different specialties including otology and endoscopic ear surgery.

5. Vesalius (Telea Electronic Engineering)[10] is a special monopolar and bipolar output device that enables the surgeon to perform surgery with an extremely delicate approach and respect of both tissues and biologic structures. Quantum Molecular Resonance is named for the particular way the energy is transferred to the biologic tissue in the form of high frequency electrical fields that interact with the tissue itself. The cutting effect does not depend on an increase of the temperature but, instead, on the breaking up of cells due to the induced resonance effect. In the cutting mode, the temperature rises to 45°C. The coagulation is also obtained by using the same resonance while the energy is transferred. Importantly, the cut is not a consequence of the high heat produced in the tissue, as happens for standard electrosurgical and radiosurgical units. Instead, it is caused by the breakage of the molecular bonds and it is, therefore, obtained without temperature rise. In fact, the temperature rise is very modest at about 63°C, which sufficient to trigger the coagulation via protein denaturation process; the cellular necrosis is avoided. As a consequence, the cut and coagulation performed by Vesalius is extremely precise, delicate, and without thermal damage. It is supplied with a different set of middle ear probes specially designed for endoscopic middle ear surgery to allow fashioning of the tympanomeatal flap and possible dissection of cholesteatoma from over ossicles and epitympanic compartments.

6. The advantages of lasers in middle ear surgery for tissue removal without mechanical trauma have long been recognized. Flexible fibers allow delivery of the laser to the recesses of the temporal bone and are now used widely in the eradication of cholesteatoma.[11,12] In current practice, the principle advantages are in eradicating cholesteatoma,[13] performing stapedotomy, and, occasionally, releasing of congenital ossicular fixation (**Fig. 6**). The KTP laser is a valuable tool in endoscopic middle ear surgery that improves the surgeon's ability to remove cholesteatoma effectively. The principle advantage of the laser is in removal of residual matrix from hidden recesses, such as the subpyramidal space or supratubal recess. Such narrow areas can be inspected effectively with angled endoscopes, but conventional dissectors and forceps do not easily permit removal of retained cholesteatoma matrix without

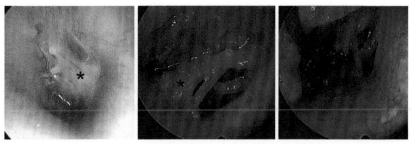

Fig. 6. Endoscopic images of congenital fixation of the left malleus handle from a tympanic bony plate (*asterisks*). KTP laser was used to free this plate from the malleus handle without torsion or mechanical displacement that could have caused cochlear injury. Four-tone average air conduction threshold improved from 41 to 18 dB HL, and bone conduction from 9 to 5 dB HL. Preoperative image, anatomic orientation (*left*). Tympanomeatal flap elevated, surgical orientation (*center*). Bony plate divided, surgical orientation (*right*). HL, hearing level.

destructive bone removal. The KTP beam can be guided into these areas because of its fine fiber carrier, which allows for disease removal by a conservative approach. Use of the laser to remove granulation tissue is of particular benefit with endoscopic surgery because bleeding into the field is minimized. Addition of the KTP laser to endoscopic middle ear surgery is expected to help reduce residual disease and improve hearing outcomes by facilitating ossicular preservation.[14] It is thus an important adjunct in the endoscopic surgeon's armamentarium.

In cholesteatoma surgery, laser is effective at ablating visible and submicroscopic remnants of cholesteatoma matrix (video 7), shrinking granulation tissue (video 8), and dividing mucosal folds (video 9). Mucosal surfaces heal well after laser has been applied to the middle ear and mastoid as shown in (**Fig. 7**). The main risk is

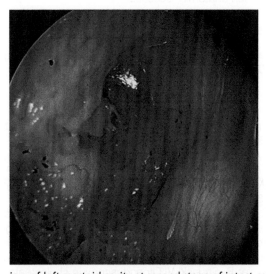

Fig. 7. Endoscopic view of left mastoid cavity at second stage of intact canal wall tympano-mastoidectomy. Specks of carbonization indicate the area where KTP laser was previously applied 1 year previously during the first stage of surgery. The mucosa and bone have healed well and the cavity is well ventilated.

inadvertent facial nerve injury[15] and, for this reason, care must be taken not to apply laser energy close to the nerve.

Practical points to consider when using KTP laser in the middle ear include the following:

- KTP is transmitted by a fiber that can be used alongside the endoscope. The fiber is slightly flexible so the tip can be adjusted for use with angled endoscopes.
- A filter can be placed in front of the camera, which filters the burst of light that would otherwise obscure the view.
- Atraumatic removal of granulation tissue, matrix, and perimatrix from ossicular chain is possible.[16] It is claimed that it is less damaging to cochlea than mechanical dissection of ossicles.[12]
- A power setting of 1 W can be used with a defocused beam to paint areas where cholesteatoma is adherent to reduce the presence of submicroscopic deposits of residual cholesteatoma (not near the facial nerve).
- Lower power settings are effective at ablating residual matrix from the ossicles (300–400 mW).
- Smoke does not need clearing with two handed microscope-guided surgery. In one-handed endoscope-guided surgery, an assistant can hold a sucker in the meatus (although this is simplest, it can be awkward, and there is danger of accidental advancement of the sucker into the stapes); or attach it to the endoscope or the laser probe with Steristrips.[17]

SUMMARY

State-of-the-art devices and instruments have been specially designated for endoscopic ear surgery, contributing to the progress of the specialty. These instruments help expand the indications and refine the surgical skills for this surgery, allowing better control of pathological conditions and permitting access to previously unreachable or difficult to reach anatomic recesses.

SUPPLEMENTARY DATA

Supplementary data related to this article are found online at http://dx.doi.org/10.1016/j.otc.2012.10.005.

REFERENCES

1. Tarabichi M. Transcanal endoscopic management of cholesteatoma. Otol Neurotol 2010;31:580–8.
2. Thomassin JM, Korchia D, Doris JM. Endoscopic-guided oto-surgery in the prevention of residual cholesteatoma. Laryngoscope 1883;103:939–43.
3. Badr-El-Dine M. Value of ear endoscopy in cholesteatoma surgery. Otol Neurotol 2002;23:631–5.
4. El-Meselaty K, Badr-El-Dine M, Mandour M, et al. Endoscope affects decision making in cholesteatoma surgery. Otolaryngol Head Neck Surg 2003;129:490–6.
5. Presuti L, Marchioni D, Mattioli F, et al. Endoscopic management of acquired cholesteatoma: our experience. Otolaryngol Head Neck Surg 2008;37:1–7.
6. Ayache S, Tramier B, Strunski V. Otoendoscopy in cholesteatoma surgery of the middle ear. What benefits can be expected? Otol Neurotol 2008;29:1085–90.
7. Marchioni D, Mattioli F, Alicandri-Ciufelli M, et al. Trans-canal endoscopic approach to the sinus tympani: a clinical report. Otol Neurotol 2009;30:758–65.

8. Badr-El-Dine M, El-Garem HF, Talaat AM, et al. Endoscopically assisted minimally invasive microvascular decompression of hemifacial spasm. Otol Neurotol 2002; 23:122–8.
9. Piezosurgery Medical manufactured by Mectron medical technology. Genoa (Italy): Peizosurgery S.R.L. Available at: www.piezosurgery.com.
10. VESALIUS MC bipolar coagulation/cutting device. By Telea Electronic Engineering. Vicenza (Italy). Available at: www.vesalius.it; www.teleamedical.com.
11. Kakehata S, Futai K, Kuroda R, et al. Office-based endoscopic procedure for diagnosis in conductive hearing loss cases using OtoScan laser-assisted myringotomy. Laryngoscope 2004;114:1285–9.
12. Saeed SR, Jackler RK. Lasers in surgery for chronic ear disease. Otolaryngol Clin North Am 1996;29:245–56.
13. Hamilton JW. Efficacy of the KTP laser in the treatment of middle ear cholesteatoma. Otol Neurotol 2005;26:135–9.
14. James A. Ossicular preservation in paediatric cholesteatoma: the contribution of laser and endoscopic surgery. in press.
15. Eskander A, Holler T, Papsin BC. Delayed facial nerve paresis after using the KTP laser in the treatment of cholesteatoma despite inter-operative facial nerve monitoring. Int J Pediatr Otorhinolaryngol 2010;74:823–4.
16. Hamilton JW. Systematic preservation of the ossicular chain in cholesteatoma surgery using a fiber-guided laser. Otol Neurotol 2010;31:1104–8.
17. Clark MP, Commins D. One-handed KTP laser application with suction, for ear surgery. Ann R Coll Surg Engl 2006;88:500.

Transtympanic Endoscopy for Diagnosis of Middle Ear Pathology

Seiji Kakehata, MD, PhD

KEYWORDS

- Endoscopy • Transtympanic • Presurgical diagnosis • Ossicular disruption
- Laser-assisted myringotomy

KEY POINTS

- An endoscopic transtympanic procedure using laser-assisted myringotomy is a direct and reliable preoperative diagnostic method for abnormalities of the middle ear.
- This procedure is less painful and safe, and is easily performed even in young children in the outpatient clinic.
- This procedure can reveal minor anomalies around the incudostapedial joint and the superstructure of the stapes, which cannot be detected with standard high-resolution computed tomography.
- This procedure can be also applied to diagnose stapes fixation and perilymphatic fistula, which could not be diagnosed presurgically and for which exploratory tympanotomy has been necessary to make a definite diagnosis.
- This procedure offers better surgical indications and patient consultation, and is a potential alternative to exploratory tympanotomy.

 A video on transtympanic endoscopy for diagnosis of abnormalities of the middle ear accompanies this article at http://www.oto.theclinics.com/

OVERVIEW

To make a diagnosis of abnormality of the middle ear in a case of an intact tympanic membrane, exploratory tympanotomy has been necessary even when high-resolution computed tomography (CT) is applied to evaluate the condition of the middle ear. Office-based transtympanic endoscopy through the perforation made by laser-assisted myringotomy (LAM) has been introduced for the diagnosis of ossicular interruption[1], stapes fixation, tympanosclerosis, congenital cholesteatoma, and perilymphatic fistula. This procedure is effective and safe, and is a potential alternative to exploratory tympanotomy.

Department of Otolaryngology Head and Neck Surgery, Yamagata University Faculty of Medicine, 2-2-2 Iidanishi, Yamagata-shi 990-9585, Japan
E-mail address: kakehata@med.id.yamagata-u.ac.jp

Otolaryngol Clin N Am 46 (2013) 227–232
http://dx.doi.org/10.1016/j.otc.2012.10.006
0030-6665/13/$ – see front matter © 2013 Elsevier Inc. All rights reserved.

PREOPERATIVE PLANNING
Otoscopic Examination and Hearing Tests

A detailed otoscopic examination and precise hearing tests including audiometry, tympanometry, and auditory reflex are performed to make a diagnosis of a conductive hearing loss.

High-Resolution CT

High-resolution CT is applied to evaluate the condition of the ossicular chain, and the presence of the sclerotic foci, new bone formation, or cholesteatoma. However, the integrity of the ossicular chain and stapes superstructure are not optimally depicted at CT with image reconstruction in the standard axial and coronal planes. Small anatomic details of the ossicular chain, such as lack or subluxation of the incudosta-pedial (IS) joint or the interruption between crus and footplate, are very difficult to evaluate. In addition, stapes fixation has not to date been diagnosed presurgically.

A Set of Endoscopes

Rigid endoscopes with 0°, 30°, or 70° viewing angles (1.9 mm in the outer diameter; Storz, Tuttlingen, Germany) are used (**Fig. 1**). Images are delivered to a monitor through a high-definition charge-coupled device camera (Storz) attached to the endoscope lens, and recorded.

Position of Patients

The patient sits on the examination chair and is asked for the head to remain still when the endoscope is in use. The patients are also told to watch the monitor, which helps to reduce accidental movements. In the case of young children, the head is held steady by a nurse with the parent standing by.

DIAGNOSTIC TECHNIQUES AND PROCEDURES
Laser-Assisted Myringotomy

In the outpatient clinic, a circular perforation with a diameter of 2 mm is made in the tympanic membrane with a CO_2 laser unit (OtoLAM; Lumenis, Yokneam, Israel) after

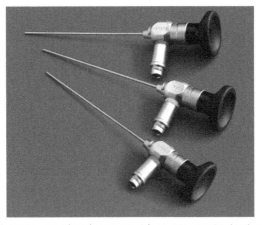

Fig. 1. A set of endoscopes. Rigid endoscopes with 0°, 30°, or 70° viewing angles (1.9 mm in the outer diameter; Storz, Germany). (*Courtesy of* Karl Storz GmbH & Co. KG, Tuttlingen, Germany; with permission.)

tympanic membrane anesthesia using iontophoresis. The location of the perforation is between the oval window and the round window (**Fig. 2**). A single pulse of 10 W is used; if this is insufficient, a subsequent pulse of 10 W or less is made. LAM provides a bloodless circular perforation, and an endoscope inserted through the perforation provides a clear view of the middle ear. A perforation with a diameter of less than 2 mm is closed within 2 to 3 weeks.

Endoscopy of the Middle Ear

0°, 30°, or 70° rigid endoscopes are advanced slowly toward the perforation. Endoscopic views through endoscopes held immediately to the outer side of the myringotomy perforation provide clear views of the mesotympanum (**Fig. 3**). When necessary, the tip of the endoscope is inserted into the tympanic cavity through the nonhemorrhagic perforation. The endoscopy is begun with a 0°degree endoscope to obtain a feel for proper positioning of the endoscope, and then proceeds to 30° and 70° endoscopes. Insertion of the scopes passing through the perforation into the mesotympanum permits close-up views of the stapes and, especially when using a 70° endoscope, further inspection of the epitympanum. The incus body, isthmus of the tympani, and chorda tympani are clearly visible through a 70° endoscope. In the case of a 70° endoscope, introduction to the perforation needs additional care because front visualization is lacking.

Ossicular interruption

A nonhemorrhagic, round perforation permits clear views of the IS joint with a 30° endoscope. This scope clearly reveals disruption of the ossicular chain, connective tissue strand replacing long process, absence of IS joint, hypoplasia of stapedial crus and lenticular process of incus, subluxation of the IS joint, or interruption between crus and footplate (**Fig. 4**). Some of these minor anomalies cannot be detected with a standard high-resolution CT scan. Transtympanic endoscopy is also applied to the treatment of conductive hearing loss, ossicular reconstruction, and removal of early congenital or recurrent pearl cholesteatomas.[2]

Stapes fixation

Stapes mobility is one of the keys to successful tympanoplasty. However, stapes mobility cannot be diagnosed presurgically, and exploratory tympanotomy is necessary to make a definite diagnosis of stapes fixation. To diagnose stapes fixation in the outpatient clinic, mobility of the stapes responding to the contralateral sound is

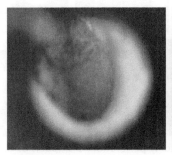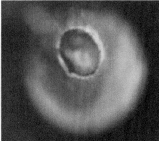

Fig. 2. Laser-assisted myringotomy. A circular perforation with a diameter of 2 mm is made in the tympanic membrane with a CO_2 laser unit between the oval window and the round window.

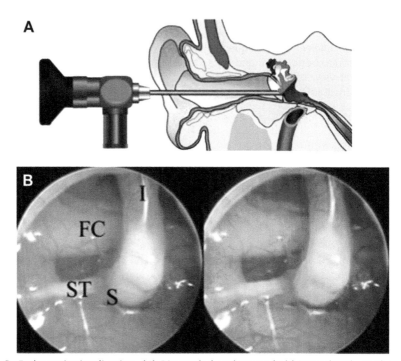

Fig. 3. Endoscopic visualization. (*A*) 30° angled endoscope held immediately to the outer side of the perforation. (*B*) Intact ossicular chain. FC, facial canal; I, incus; S, stapes; ST, stapedial tendon.

examined directly under endoscopic visualization through the perforation made by LAM.[3] The stapes reflex by contralateral stimulation is clearly observed under direct endoscopic view, and the mobility of the stapes is confirmed without touching the ear ossicles or tympanic membrane (Video 1).

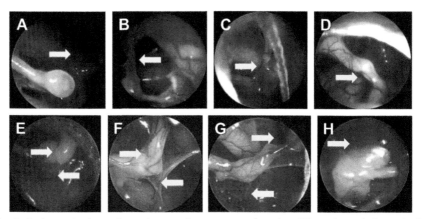

Fig. 4. Endoscopic views through a myringotomy perforation. Disruption of the ossicular chain (*A–H*), connective tissue strand replacing long process (*B, C, D*), absence of IS joint (*A–D, H*), hypoplasia of stapedial crus (*E, F*), subluxation of IS joint (*E, F, G*), or interruption between crus and footplate (*G*) were detected (*arrows*).

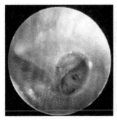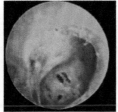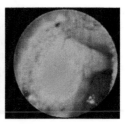

Fig. 5. Laser-assisted myringotomy. Cholesteatoma formed a circular shape and involved the superstructure of stapes.

Congenital cholesteatoma

This procedure can also be applied to diagnose congenital cholesteatoma of the open and/or closed type, with or without ossicular chain interruption. **Fig. 5** shows a case of unexpected conductive hearing loss. Otoscopic examination did not demonstrate hindrance factors such as effusion and cholesteatoma. Endoscopy of the middle ear through LAM revealed that the cholesteatoma formed a circular shape and involved the superstructure of stapes. After this examination, tympanoplasty was performed at a later date.

Perilymphatic fistula

Endoscopy of the middle ear through LAM can be applied for the diagnosis of perilymphatic fistula that could not be diagnosed presurgically. Video 2 clearly reveals fluctuating fluid around the round window and granulation tissues around the stapes.

DISCUSSION

The endoscopic procedure using LAM has several advantages. First, LAM provides a temporary bloodless circular perforation, which allows a clear view of the middle ear. The perforation is closed within about 2 weeks when the diameter of the perforation is 2 mm. Scar formation is rare, and the LAM procedure is repeatable. Second, round perforation permits inspection of abnormalities of the middle ear with the endoscopes held immediately to the outer side of the perforation. This approach is less painful and safe, and is easily performed even in young children in the outpatient clinic.

SUMMARY

An endoscopic transtympanic procedure using LAM is a direct and reliable preoperative diagnostic method for abnormalities of the middle ear, offering better surgical indications and patient consultation.

SUPPLEMENTARY DATA

Supplementary data related to this article can be found online at http://dx.doi.org/10.1016/j.otc.2012.10.006.

REFERENCES

1. Kakehata S, Futai K, Kuroda R, et al. Office-based endoscopic procedure for diagnosis in conductive hearing loss cases utilizing Otoscan laser-assisted myringotomy. Laryngoscope 2004;114:1285–9.

2. Kakehata S, Futai K, Sasaki A, et al. Endoscopic transtympanic tympanoplasty in the treatment of conductive hearing loss: early results. Otol Neurotol 2006;27:14–9.
3. Kakehata S, Kitani R, Futai K, et al. Office-based endoscopic procedure for diagnosis of stapes mobility using Otoscan laser-assisted myringotomy. The 27th Politzer Society Meeting. London, September 3–5, 2009.

Endoscopic Middle Ear Surgery in Children

Adrian L. James, MA, DM, FRCS(ORL-HNS)

KEYWORDS

- Middle ear surgery • Pediatric otology • Cholesteatoma • Tympanoplasty

KEY POINTS

- Permeatal access to middle ear is restricted by the narrower width, but facilitated by the shorter length in younger children.
- In many cases it is the curvature of the ear canal instead of the age of the child that governs endoscopic access. Totally endoscopic middle ear surgery can be completed successfully, even in infancy.
- Endoscopic visualization of the recesses of the middle ear allows a less invasive canal wall up approach that is ideally suited to children.
- The retrotympanum is a common location for cholesteatoma in children and benefits from endoscopic removal.
- Residual cholesteatoma rates can be reduced with endoscopic inspection and dissection.
- Removal of cholesteatoma from the medial epitympanum can be completed endoscopically without disarticulating an intact ossicular chain and so improve hearing outcome.

 Videos of Endoscopic Techniques in Children accompany this article

INTRODUCTION

The wide-angle view from the tip of a rigid endoscope provides advantages to the otologist in many aspects of pediatric care, ranging from assessment of the ear drum in clinic to minimally invasive access to the hidden recesses of the temporal bone during surgery. In clinic, the recording of endoscopic images improves accuracy in monitoring changes in tympanic membrane retraction.[1] In surgery, endoscopes are used for inspection (eg, to reveal occult remnants of cholesteatoma) but, more importantly, they can be used with angled instruments and laser to remove disease from under hidden recesses without destructive bone removal. The child benefits from the consequent reduction in residual cholesteatoma[2] and gain in hearing from more frequent ossicular preservation.[3] An intact canal wall approach is generally favored for pediatric cholesteatoma surgery[4] and the endoscope is an invaluable asset in the combined

The author has no financial associations with industry or other conflicts of interest.
Department of Otolaryngology—Head and Neck Surgery, Hospital for Sick Children, University of Toronto, 555 University Avenue, Toronto, Ontario M5G 1X8, Canada
E-mail address: adr.james@utoronto.ca

Otolaryngol Clin N Am 46 (2013) 233–244
http://dx.doi.org/10.1016/j.otc.2012.10.007
0030-6665/13/$ – see front matter © 2013 Elsevier Inc. All rights reserved.

approach through ear canal and mastoid. Although access is more challenging in the smaller pediatric ear canal, totally endoscopic middle ear surgery through the canal is still appropriate in many cases, avoiding the disadvantage to the child of an external incision. The opportunities and methods for application of endoscopes to pediatric middle ear surgery are outlined in this article.

The principle advantage of a totally endoscopic surgical approach for the child is avoidance of an external incision. For the surgeon, the avoidance of a small endaural incision or of a cosmetically placed incision just behind the postauricular sulcus might seem a small advantage. However, the universal expression of relief and pleasure on the faces of parents and children on learning that it has been possible to avoid an external incision indicates that this is perceived as a significant benefit by the patient. In addition to the psychological and cosmetic benefits, more tangible advantages include the possibility of a shorter hospital stay (same day discharge can be anticipated) and faster return to the physical sports in which many children participate. These benefits are outweighed by the principles of achieving a safe dry ear, and the functional importance of an intact tympanic membrane and ossicular chain. Therefore, selection of a totally endoscopic permeatal approach has to be considered carefully and not allowed to compromise the primary objectives of surgery.

The advantages to the otologist of endoscopy are clearly demonstrated throughout this issue and center around the panoramic view of the middle ear cleft that endoscopy provides. The extent to which an endoscope is used in the ear of a child depends not just on the condition of that child's ear but also on the availability of resource and experience of the otologist. With appropriate circumstances, a full range of otologic procedures can be completed in part or totally with endoscopy. The tools required are, in the main, no different from those used in adults because the middle ear and tympanic membrane approximate to adult size at birth.[5] By starting with sinonasal endoscopes and conventional middle ear instruments, the surgeon can gradually develop the skills and experience that may then justify procurement of more specialized instruments. These in turn will facilitate development of greater expertise. So, although in the first instance the endoscope may simply be used for inspection in clinic or intraoperatively, with time it will supplement, and in some cases ultimately supplant, the microscope for pediatric middle ear surgery. This article is based on experience using the endoscope increasingly in pediatric middle ear surgery over the last decade and outlines the potential scope of pediatric otoendoscopic practice, steps for appropriate case selection, procedural tips for children's ears, and discussion of the place of endoscopy in comparison with microscopy in pediatric ear surgery.

RANGE OF ENDOSCOPIC INTERVENTIONS

It is conceivable that the scope of endoscopic applications in pediatric otologic practice will increase in the future. A wide range of interventions is currently available.

Preoperative and Postoperative Assessment

Short (6 cm) rigid endoscopes are very useful for image-capture for patient and parental education, monitoring tympanic membrane retraction, and for careful preoperative planning. Insufflation adapters allow endoscopic assessment of adherence of retracted areas (**Fig. 1**, Video 1). The clearer optics of the 4 mm scope are preferable for most children, though the 2.7 mm scope is occasionally necessary for the narrower meatus of young children. Although angled endoscopes can help to visualize the depths of a retraction pocket, in practice it can be difficult to get the endoscope sufficiently close to a child's tympanic membrane to be able to see deeply into a pocket.

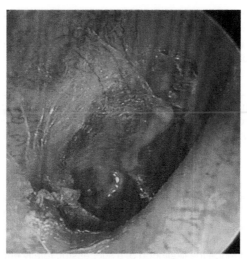

Fig. 1. Endoscopic video of the right tympanic membrane during insufflation of the ear canal. Part of the retracted pars tensa elevates with reduction in ear canal air pressure, but a section remains adherent to the promontory by the round window niche. Of note, the deeply retracted pars flaccida is not mobile, consistent with the different ventilation pathways and mechanisms of disease in pars flaccida retraction and cholesteatoma. (*Data from* Marchioni D, Alicandri-Ciufelli M, Molteni G, et al. Selective epitympanic dysventilation syndrome. Laryngoscope 2010;120:1028.)

Any skin contact of the endoscope within the bony meatus is painful and likely to preclude further cooperation.

Intraoperative Inspection

The rigid endoscope is used by many otologists to inspect the retrotympanum or other hidden areas after microscope-guided dissection of cholesteatoma. This intervention has the potential to lower residual disease rates significantly.[6,7] For thorough inspection, curved suckers must be used to clear blood from these areas.

Tube Insertion

Endoscopy provides excellent visualization for tube insertion, which is helpful for teaching and in settings in which a microscope is not available (Video 2). It is not practical in the youngest or syndromic children with narrow ear canals.

Tympanotomy

Elevation of a tympanomeatal flap and insertion of an angled endoscope provides a good view of the middle ear cleft and under the ossicular chain for assessment of conductive hearing loss and residual cholesteatoma. The availability of thin, angled endoscopes (eg, 1.7 mm 30°) makes it possible to achieve limited inspection of the middle ear cleft though a myringotomy.

Tympanoplasty and Cholesteatoma

The full range of tympanoplasty techniques is used in pediatric tympanoplasty.[8] A simple patch myringoplasty or a butterfly graft is ideal for tympanostomy tube site perforations. Underlay or lateral onlay techniques can both be completed endoscopically for larger pediatric perforations. The endoscope is especially beneficial in surgery for tympanic membrane atelectasis because direct visualization for elevation of the retraction from the retrotympanum is provided.

As foreseen by Tarabichi,[9] the endoscopic approach remains most valuable in tympanoplasty and cholesteatoma surgery (see later discussion).

Other

Petrous apex lesions and perilymph leak are rare in children but can be approached endoscopically. Endoscopic visualization of the Eustachian tube[10] and cochlea[11] may prove valuable in future.

CASE SELECTION

As in all aspects of surgery, good results can only be anticipated from appropriate case selection. It can be hard to determine preoperatively whether an entirely endoscopic approach will be possible, or even appropriate, in any given pediatric patient. Therefore, it is important to obtain consent for an external incision in case it is needed. Several variables influence the likelihood of a successful, totally endoscopic approach.

Morphology of the External Auditory Meatus

The width, length, and tortuosity of the ear canal, particularly the bony portion, determine the feasibility of endoscopic access. A meatus narrower than the 4.5 mm speculum is likely to resist an endoscopic permeatal approach. The bony meatus is narrower in young children, restricting access for instruments alongside the endoscope; however, it is also shorter, which increases the angulation and range of movement achievable. A deep anterior recess or prominent hump on floor of meatus can significantly impede access, though bone can be removed with curettage to improve access if necessary. Piezoelectric bone removal may prove effective (see the article by Badr-El-Dine and colleagues elsewhere in this issue), but drilling of bone is limited by the challenges of clearing irrigation fluid and spray. As shown in (**Fig. 2**), individual configuration of these proportions is more important than age in determining access and totally endoscopic middle ear surgery can be completed successfully even in infancy. The author's personal experience includes, for example, the identification and successful patching of a traumatic round window perilymph leak in a two-and-one-half year old child totally endoscopically (Video 3).

Indication for Surgery

As in adults, the commonest applications for endoscopic middle ear surgery are likely to be in tympanic membrane perforation and acquired cholesteatoma.[9] Acquired cholesteatoma commonly arises from the pars tensa in children (**Fig. 3**), more so than in adults.[12] Therefore, it frequently extends into the retrotympanum. Cholesteatoma in this area is ideally suited to endoscopic surgery.[13–15] However pediatric cholesteatoma more commonly extends deeply into the mastoid,[12] beyond the limits of what is readily achievable with a totally endoscopic permeatal approach. Canal wall up surgery is widely favored in children[4] and an endoscopic permeatal canal wall down approach to pediatric cholesteatoma would not currently seem an appropriate option. So, if cholesteatoma can be removed via an endoscopic permeatal atticoantrostomy, reconstruction of the canal wall defect with cartilage would be appropriate. The size of canal defect achievable with curettage endoscopically is likely to be adequately covered by a tragal graft. Larger cholesteatomas still require an open approach with drilling of the mastoid cortex.

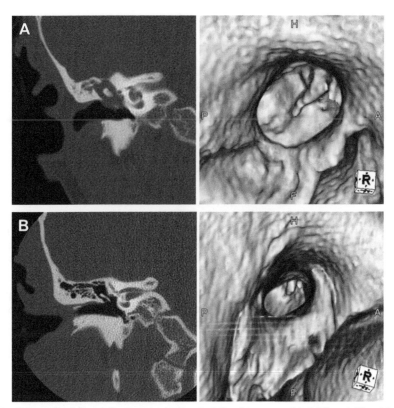

Fig. 2. CT images of the right temporal bone in (*A*) a four-year-old child and (*B*) a 14-year-old child. Left panels show coronal sections through the ear canal. Right panels show multiplanar reconstruction looking through the canal to the malleus handle. The ear canal of the younger child is clearly shorter, which allows good freedom of movement for instruments in permeatal surgery. Uncharacteristically, the canal is narrower in the older child, showing that the proportions of the individual are more important than age in determining feasibility of permeatal endoscopic access.

When congenital cholesteatoma is detected sufficiently early, it may be confined to the mesotympanum and supratubal recess, or extend a short distance into the medial epitympanum (**Fig. 4**). A totally endoscopic permeatal approach is ideally suited to such lesions. Placement of an angled endoscope in the anteroinferior mesotympanum provides visualization for access to the supratubal recess and anterior surface of the processus cochleariformis from which congenital cholesteatoma most commonly arises (Video 4). Long, angled instruments or the KTP laser may be necessary for removal of matrix from these sites without disruption of the ossicular chain (Video 5).[3]

The use of endoscopy for staged second-look procedures has been advocated.[16,17] This is certainly feasible for disease that was entirely accessible through the ear canal initially. However, access to the mastoid via a small stab incision is unlikely to provide adequate visualization of occult residual disease in many cases because of the tendency of the mastoid cortex to regrow in children, and because the cavity is often filled with obstructive scar tissue. Although ossiculoplasty can be completed endoscopically, precise positioning of total ossicular replacement prostheses is challenging with a one-handed technique, especially within the confines of a pediatric

Site of origin of pediatric cholesteatoma

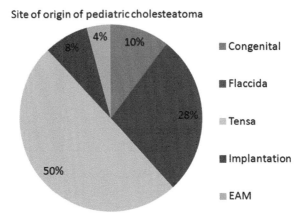

- ■ Congenital
- ■ Flaccida
- ▨ Tensa
- ■ Implantation
- ▨ EAM

Fig. 3. Proportion of cholesteatomas arising at different locations. In contrast to adult series, pars tensa cholesteatoma is nearly twice as common as that arising from the pars flaccida. Prospectively acquired data from a consecutive series of 267 children with cholesteatoma at the Hospital for Sick children. (*Data from* James, 2012, unpublished data.)

meatus. With an intact stapes and eroded incus, the author favors cartilage tympanoplasty over incus interposition or partial ossicular replacement prosthesis, to achieve good hearing results and prevent recurrence of pars tensa retraction.[18]

Extent of Pathologic State

When considering a totally endoscopic approach for repair of tympanic membrane defects (with or without cholesteatoma) the location of the perforation must be considered in relation to the tortuosity of the ear canal, regarding ease of access. Also, the size of the child's tragus must be compared with the size of the perforation, with edges stripped, if tragal perichondrium or cartilage is to be used for the repair becauses it may be too small to close a large perforation. Consent for use of other donor sites or materials would then be required.

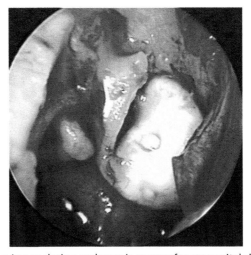

Fig. 4. Intraoperative image during endoscopic surgery for congenital cholesteatoma of the right ear. The tympanic membrane has been elevated off the malleus handle to provide access for removal of the lesion.

Size and location of the lesion are also important considerations when planning totally endoscopic cholesteatoma surgery. False negative and false positive identification occurs with CT and MRI so these devices cannot always predict the extent of the disease. Completion of a totally endoscopic approach when the child and parents are prepared for an external approach will be welcomed more warmly than the opposite scenario! Although pediatric cholesteatoma has a reputation for being more extensive than adult disease, the condition certainly can be detected while still small and, in the author's region, a high proportion are localized only to the epitympanum and meso-tympanum within reach of totally endoscopic access.[3,4]

Reconstruction

Before embarking on a totally endoscopic approach to cholesteatoma or perforation, consideration must be given to the method of tympanic membrane reconstruction. The tragus is the optimum donor site for endoscopic ear surgery because the incision for access can be hidden on the posterior surface. Although the tympanic membrane approximates to adult size at birth, the tragus is considerably smaller in children, so it may prove may be inadequate for larger perforations. If a larger graft is required than that provided by the tragus, consent for an alternative graft may be required (see later discussion). Furthermore, use of an external incision reduces the principle benefit of the incisionless permeatal approach: use of a postaural or endaural incision for access and donor site should be considered, with or without the benefit of an endoscope.

TECHNICAL TIPS FOR ENDOSCOPIC PEDIATRIC MIDDLE EAR SURGERY

Although the principles and specifics of the endoscopic approach to the ear are the same of children and adults, the following points are considered especially pertinent to the application of this technique to children.

1. Reduce bleeding. This is one of the highest priorities in endoscopic middle ear surgery.
    a. Canal infiltration. Injection of bupivicaine with 1:200,000 adrenaline helps to reduce bleeding. 1:100,000 adrenaline solution has been reported to cause transient tachycardia without any less bleeding in adult sinus surgery[19]; therefore, it is perhaps better avoided in children's surgery. A better view is achieved by slow injection so as to avoid blebbing and minimize the number of puncture sites because these bleed slightly. Infiltration of the superior canal wall is easiest because the skin is thicker and not adherent to the tympanic ring, but the most attention is required where a flap is to be raised.
    b. Care to avoid abrasion of the meatal skin with the tip or shaft of endoscope or instruments is of importance in the narrow pediatric meatus.
    c. Controlled hypotension. Successful completion of tympanoplasty and suban-nular tube insertion has been reported in children under local anesthesia.[20,21] However, in the author's practice to date, children receive general anesthesia. Communication with the anesthetist to provide optimal conditions is important. Anecdotally, a heart rate of less than or equal to 80 beats per minute and blood pressure in the order of 80/35 mm Hg generally seem to provide good conditions. The services of a pediatric anesthetist help to ensure that this is done safely.
    d. Epinephrine-soaked cotton balls. Cotton wool balls can be trimmed for small spaces and unlike synthetic foam, conform to the required shape. They are useful for retraction of the tympanomeatal skin flap (either under it to push it away from the bone or placed on the everted edge of the flap).

e. Bleeding generally becomes less of a problem once the drum has been lifted. In some cases significant patience with control of bleeding is required to get to this point.

2. Shave hairs. The hairs of even young children may extend well into the narrow pediatric external auditory meatus (EAM). The clarity of the visual field is easily impaired by a smearing of the smallest trace of wax or blood from these hairs across the lens of the endoscope as it is passed into the ear. Rudimentary trimming of these hairs (eg, with small curved iris scissors) minimizes this problem. There is no need to shave them flush to the skin (eg, with a scalpel) because resultant skin abrasion may provide an additional of source of bleeding into the field.

3. Choice of endoscopes. For many surgeons, this may be limited by the range of scopes available in the operating room for other purposes. Resources allowing, a full selection of 0°, 30°, 45°, and 70° scopes of different diameters might be ideal, but few would be used regularly. As a minimum, a 4 mm 0° scope is good for initial assessment of the tympanic membrane and will allow adequate access for raising the tympanomeatal flap in most children. For surgery within the mesotympanum and epitympanum, a narrower angled scope is required. The 30° 2.7 mm scope is effective, but the newer 3 mm scopes have vastly superior optics for illumination and clarity. A 45° angle generally provides a more useful field of view for retrotympanic and epitympanic access. A 70° scope is occasionally useful for examining the under surfaces of structures such as the medial surface of the incus though the tympanic recess or the medial surface of the pyramidal eminence in the subpyramidal recess. Unlike the 30° and 45° scopes, the 70° does not give a view of structures lying directly in front of the tip of the scope so extra care is required to avoid ossicular trauma. Optimal length of the endoscope is between 11 and 20 cm, according to the surgeon's preference. If it is too short, movement of instruments is impaired by the head of the scope and camera; if it is too long, it becomes difficult to stabilize the scope.

4. Additional instrumentation. Acquisition of dedicated equipment can transform the surgeon's ability to complete pediatric surgery endoscopically. The following have been found to be very beneficial:
   a. Curved or angled instruments (eg, Thomassin set, Storz, Germany)
   b. KTP laser plus filter (see the article by Badr-El-Dine and colleagues elsewhere in this issue)
   c. High-definition camera and monitor.

5. Stabilizing the endoscope. It is generally easier for the surgeon to hold the endoscope instead of using an assistant or mechanical scope holder for the following reasons, which are especially relevant in the smaller pediatric ear:
   a. Movement of the scope allows the surgeon to optimize his or her view for the specific task in hand.
   b. The position of the scope can be adjusted to follow safe insertion and removal of instruments from the ear, and to allow optimum angulation and movement of instruments within the ear.
   c. It is likely that the surgeon's ability to associate proprioceptive feedback from small movements of the scope with corresponding changes in the field of view aids three-dimensional appreciation of the anatomy. This sensory feedback may be particularly advantageous in the small confines of the middle ear cleft in comparison, for example, with endoscopic anterior skull base surgery in which a four-handed approach is often used.
   d. Two-point stabilization of the scope helps to give a very stable visual field. The shaft of the scope rests firmly on the side of the opening of the EAM. The

surgeon's elbow or forearm can be rested on the arm or back rest of the chair or on an adjustable stand. It should be noted that too much pressure from the surgeon's arm resting on the chest of a child can increase bleeding by obstructing venous return.[22]

6. Tympanic membrane reconstruction.

The tragus provides the optimum donor site for perichondrium or cartilage because the incision for access is well hidden within the meatus. Both cartilage and perichondrium are thinner and more delicate than in adults, so additional care is required to avoid damage during harvest. The cartilage is often an optimal thickness for tensa reconstruction without the need for shaving. The curve of superior edge of the tragus often matches the curve of the posterior annulus. This is ideal for reconstruction: if intact perichondrium is harvested on both sides of the graft, it can reflect off the convex (usually the anterior) surface and kept in continuity around the superior edge of the graft. Perichondrium can then be draped up the posterior wall of the EAM so providing good stability for the graft.

Other autografts: other donor sites can be used, though this does reduce the benefit of having no external incision that is otherwise achievable with a totally endoscopic approach.

Other materials: Allograft (eg, AlloDerm; LifeCell Corporation, Branchburg, NJ, USA), xenograft (eg, Gelfoam; Pfizer Inc, New York, NY, USA), or synthetic materials (eg, Epidisk; Medtronic Xomed Inc, Jacksonville, FL, USA) may be used as adjuncts to facilitate or support tympanic membrane repair without recourse to an external incision. Of these, AlloDerm in particular can be used for reconstruction of larger defects or revision surgery after previous use of the tragus as a donor site.

TOTALLY ENDOSCOPIC OR ENDOSCOPE-ASSISTED MIDDLE EAR SURGERY?

As stated in the introduction, the extent to which individual surgeons choose to use the endoscope in pediatric middle ear surgery will depend on several factors. The surgeon's training, preference, and experience are the most influential factors. Some surgeons rely predominantly on the endoscope alone in children as well as in adults. Currently, the author predominantly prefers to use both the endoscope and microscope in most middle ear surgery and switches from one to the other according to need. Occasional cases, such as tympanoplasty or exploratory tympanotomy, are performed endoscopically without availability of the microscope. The endoscope is almost always used for dissection of tympanic retraction or cholesteatoma from out of the retrotympanum (Video 6). In this area it is vastly superior to the microscope (Video 7) and can help to significantly reduce the likelihood of residual disease in this otherwise challenging area.[2] Excessive bleeding or an unusually tortuous meatus are the only barriers to the benefits of endoscopy at this site. Endoscopy is nearly always used in preference to the microscope for clearance of cholesteatoma from underneath an intact ossicular chain, either through the ear canal, through the mastoid, or both. A two-handed approach with the microscope is easier when drilling bone to clear irrigation fluid and bone dust, so the microscope is usually used when a magnified view is needed in the mastoid. However, even within the mastoid the endoscope can provide advantages over the microscope in providing a more complete view (**Fig. 5**). An anteriorly-placed sigmoid in a typically sclerotic pediatric mastoid can block the straight-line view required for microscopy; therefore, endoscopy can be invaluable when removing cholesteatoma from the medial epitympanum under intact ossicles or from a deep sinus tympani via the retrofacial approach (**Fig. 6**; Videos 8 and 9). Although total ossicular replacement is possible endoscopically, it is

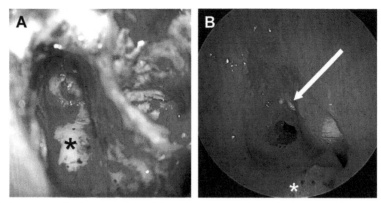

Fig. 5. Intraoperative images of the right epitympanum through the mastoid at the second stage of intact canal wall surgery. (*A*) Microscope view revealing no sign of residual cholesteatoma. (*B*) View with 45° endoscope revealing pearl of residual cholesteatoma above the superior wall of the ear canal (*arrow*). The undersurface of the tympanic membrane cartilage graft is also seen. An asterisk marks the same location on the lateral semicircular canal in both images.

often much easier to obtain optimal prosthesis or graft placement with two hands. It can be advantageous to have a microscope available for this purpose, depending on the surgeon's experience with endoscopy.

In summary, availability of both endoscopy and microscopy for most cases is advisable in pediatric middle ear surgery until confidence from an adequate experience with endoscopy has been achieved. This allows the advantages of each tool to be used when required. In the experience of most surgeons that use endoscopy in the middle ear, reliance on the microscope for middle ear surgery decreases with increased endoscopic experience.

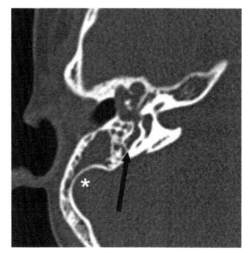

Fig. 6. Axial CT scan of the right temporal bone. Deep extension of cholesteatoma between the posterior semicircular canal and facial nerve (*arrow*). The sigmoid sinus (*asterisk*) limits retrofacial access with the microscope, but not the endoscope.

SUMMARY

The endoscope is of great value in pediatric middle ear surgery. It has clear advantages over the microscope for visualization and instrumentation in the hidden recesses of the retrotympanum and medial epitympanum that have long been recognized.[23,24] It facilitates more conservative surgery and some cases can be completed entirely endoscopically, avoiding the requirement for a postauricular incision. This is always greatly appreciated by children and their parents, and makes same-day discharge more feasible. Morphology of the pediatric ear canal and extent of disease often prevent an entirely endoscopic approach. In such cases, the endoscope is still often invaluable, allowing more frequent preservation of the ossicular chain and intact canal wall. Reduced rates of residual cholesteatoma and improved hearing thresholds can be anticipated with this approach. The learning curve for endoscopic middle ear surgery is long, even for surgeons experienced in microscope-guided middle ear surgery. Advances in instrumentation may allow more to be done more easily in future.

SUPPLEMENTARY DATA

Supplementary data related to this article can be found online at http://dx.doi.org/10.1016/j.otc.2012.10.007.

REFERENCES

1. James AL, Papsin BC, Trimble K, et al. Tympanic membrane retraction: an endoscopic evaluation of staging systems. Laryngoscope 2012;122:1115.
2. Kanotra SP, James AL. The role of endoscopy in pediatric cholesteatoma. In: Society for Ear Nose Throat Advances in Children. Kansas City, 2011.
3. James AL. Approaches to cholesteatoma with an intact ossicular chain: Combined use of microscope, endoscope and laser. In: Proceedings of the 9th International Conference on Cholesteatoma and Ear Surgery. Amsterdam: Kugler Publications; 2012.
4. Osborn AJ, Papsin BC, James AL. Clinical indications for canal wall-down mastoidectomy in a pediatric population. Otolaryngol Head Neck Surg 2012; 147:316–22.
5. Dahm MC, Shepherd RK, Clark GM. The postnatal growth of the temporal bone and its implications for cochlear implantation in children. Acta Otolaryngol Suppl 1993;505:1.
6. Good GM, Isaacson G. Otoendoscopy for improved pediatric cholesteatoma removal. Ann Otol Rhinol Laryngol 1999;108:893.
7. Kanotra SP, James AL. Otoendoscopy in the management of congenital cholesteatoma. Otolaryngol Head Neck Surg 2012;147(S2):P102.
8. James AL, Papsin BC. Ten Top Considerations in Pediatric Tympanoplasty. Otolaryngol Head Neck Surg 2012.
9. Tarabichi M. Endoscopic middle ear surgery. Ann Otol Rhinol Laryngol 1999; 108:39.
10. Grimmer JF, Poe DS. Update on eustachian tube dysfunction and the patulous eustachian tube. Curr Opin Otolaryngol Head Neck Surg 2005;13:277.
11. Manolidis S, Tonini R, Spitzer J. Endoscopically guided placement of prefabricated cochlear implant electrodes in a common cavity malformation. Int J Pediatr Otorhinolaryngol 2006;70:591.

12. Hamilton J, Rhagava N. Comparison of the characteristics of cholesteatoma at the time of surgery in children and adults. In: Ozgirgin ON, editor. Surgery of the ear——Current topics. Antalya (Turkey): Rekmay; 2009. p. 187.
13. Thomassin JM, Danvin BJ, Collin M. Endoscopic anatomy of the posterior tympanum. Rev Laryngol Otol Rhinol (Bord) 2008;129:239.
14. Marchioni D, Alicandri-Ciufelli M, Grammatica A, et al. Pyramidal eminence and subpyramidal space: an endoscopic anatomical study. Laryngoscope 2010; 120:557.
15. Marchioni D, Alicandri-Ciufelli M, Piccinini A, et al. Inferior retrotympanum revisited: an endoscopic anatomic study. Laryngoscope 2010;120:1880–6.
16. Rosenberg SI, Silverstein H, Hoffer M, et al. Use of endoscopes for chronic ear surgery in children. Arch Otolaryngol Head Neck Surg 1995;121:870.
17. Youssef TF, Poe DS. Endoscope-assisted second-stage tympanomastoidectomy. Laryngoscope 1997;107:1341.
18. Kandasamy T, James AL. Effectiveness of ossiculoplasty after erosion of the incus in children with cholesteatoma. In: Proceedings of the 9th International Conference on Cholesteatoma and Ear Surgery. Amsterdam: Kugler Publications; 2012.
19. Moshaver A, Lin D, Pinto R, et al. The hemostatic and hemodynamic effects of epinephrine during endoscopic sinus surgery: a randomized clinical trial. Arch Otolaryngol Head Neck Surg 2009;135:1005.
20. Saliba I, Boutin T, Arcand P, et al. Advantages of subannular tube vs repetitive transtympanic tube technique. Arch Otolaryngol Head Neck Surg 2011;137:1210.
21. Saliba I, Woods O. Hyaluronic acid fat graft myringoplasty: a minimally invasive technique. Laryngoscope 2011;121:375.
22. Battersby EF. Paediatric anaesthesia. In: Adams DA, Cinnamond MJ, editors. Scott-Brown's otolaryngology, vol. 6, 6th edition. Oxford (England): Butterworth-Heinemann; 1997. p. 18.
23. Thomassin JM, Korchia D, Doris JM. Endoscopic-guided otosurgery in the prevention of residual cholesteatomas. Laryngoscope 1993;103:939.
24. Bottrill ID, Poe DS. Endoscope-assisted ear surgery. Am J Otol 1995;16:158.

Introducing Endoscopic Ear Surgery into Practice

David D. Pothier, MBChB, MSc, FRCS(ORL-HNS)

KEYWORDS

- Endoscopic ear surgery • Cholesteatoma • Tympanoplasty • Minimal access

KEY POINTS

- Endoscopic ear surgery allows a minimally invasive approach to the middle ear.
- The technique has a different learning curve than traditional techniques; training is useful to allow more consistent progress when getting started.
- It can be useful to collaborate with other, more experienced surgeons who are more familiar with endoscopic ear surgery.
- A high-resolution computed tomography scan is useful before any middle ear procedure whereby the endoscopic approach is to be used.
- It is vital to discuss whether more invasive surgery may need to be undertaken should the endoscopic approach not be successful at the first instance.
- Undertaking endoscopic ear surgery through a narrow external auditory meatus can be challenging, but there are several techniques that will help considerably and allow for the wide view of the endoscope to be used to maximum advantage.

INSTRUMENTATION AND EQUIPMENT

Overview

Undertaking endoscopic ear surgery uses techniques similar to those of standard microscopic ear surgery, but does so through a very different approach to the middle ear and to abnormalities therein. The instruments required are similar to those used in standard ear surgery with the exception that certain dissectors and a forceps need to be adapted so as to take advantage of the endoscope's ability to "see round corners." The most basic instrument sets will be sufficient to undertake simple cholesteatoma and tympanoplasty surgery, but as the surgeon becomes more confident and experienced in the technique of endoscopic ear surgery, so will the requirement for more advanced tools increase.

Despite the fact that the instruments used during endoscopic middle ear surgery are very similar to those for standard ear surgery, the way in which they are used differs

Department of Otolaryngology, Head and Neck Surgery, Toronto General Hospital, University Health Network, University of Toronto, 200 Elizabeth Street, Toronto, Ontario M5G 2C4, Canada
E-mail address: mail@davepothier.com

Otolaryngol Clin N Am 46 (2013) 245–255
http://dx.doi.org/10.1016/j.otc.2012.10.009
0030-6665/13/$ – see front matter © 2013 Elsevier Inc. All rights reserved.

oto.theclinics.com

considerably. Because the entrance to the ear canal is not constrained by a speculum, the surgeon is allowed a far wider angle of approach when using instruments in the more inaccessible areas of the middle ear such as the hypotympanum or retrotympanum.

Perhaps the most major departure in technique is the one-handed nature of endoscopic ear surgery. The endoscope is held in the nondominant hand while the opposite hand undertakes the majority of the surgery. Although this seems somewhat difficult and perhaps strange at first, on analysis, the function of the nondominant hand during traditional surgery is usually to maintain suction and remove blood from the operative field while the dominant hand still undertakes the majority of the delicate surgery. Given that an endoscopic approach is considerably less traumatic than a standard approach to the middle ear, there is usually far less bleeding, so the need for suction is reduced considerably.

Choice of Endoscope

Endoscopes come in a wide array of lengths, diameters, and angles of view. Each has its own advantages and disadvantages, but the general rule is that the larger the diameter of the endoscope, the better the field of view and the better is the illumination delivered by the light bundles carried alongside the lens. As a result, a longer, wider endoscope is the preferred instrument for work in the middle ear. Most middle ear endoscopic surgeons will undertake the majority of their surgeries using a 14- to 18-cm, 3-mm diameter 0° Hopkins rod and scope (the same endoscope used for sinus surgery). In fact, it is unusual to need to change to a larger angle to achieve a good view of all of the middle ear. Sometimes, particularly in the sinus tympani, it may be necessary to change to a 30° endoscope or, even more rarely, a 45° endoscope, but this is unusual given the very wide field of view available using low-angle endoscopes. The length is important as well, given that additional endoscopes used to augment the microscopic approach to the middle ear are normally very short. An important advantage of using a longer endoscope is that the surgeon's two hands will be at different distances from the ear canal, and thus are less likely to interfere with one another during surgery (**Fig. 1**).

Although a high-quality Hopkins rod is paramount, it is also vital to ensure that the digital camera attached to the endoscope is also of very high specifications. One of the most important considerations is that the camera needs to be a 3CCD (triple charge-coupled device) camera rather than a single-chip camera. The reason for this is that single-chip cameras are prone to "red-out" when they are used in a very small area that contains areas of bleeding. Even though there is not much bleeding during endoscopic ear surgery, the field tends to get reddened; this causes complete saturation of the camera and the entire field takes on an orange hue, which makes the identification of anatomic structures very difficult. Undertaking surgery with a single-chip camera is not advisable, particularly for a beginner.

Collaboration

With the technique of endoscopic ear surgery expanding rapidly across the world of otology, it can be useful to collaborate with other, more experienced surgeons who are more familiar with this type of surgery. Although most experienced otologic surgeons will require no formal training to begin endoscopic ear surgery, attending a course on the technique can be of considerable value. Most courses are based around cadaveric dissection of fresh-frozen or partially preserved cadavers; unrestricted dissection of cadaveric specimens allows surgeons to experiment with the endoscope and gain the skills required to gain maximum benefit from the extended view that comes with an endoscopic view.

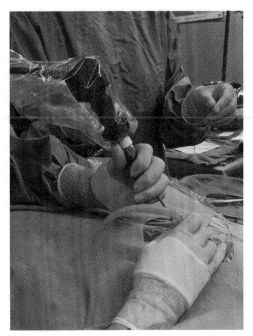

Fig. 1. Hand position.

Although getting started right away with simpler cases is perfectly reasonable, making a clinical visit to a surgeon who is already using the technique extensively can steepen the learning curve for endoscopic ear surgery. Many small technical tips can be of considerable value when undertaking endoscopic ear surgery, and these "pearls" are best learned at the elbow of an experienced surgeon who has garnered these skills over a career focused on this technique.

YOUR FIRST CASE IN ENDOSCOPIC EAR SURGERY

When starting out with endoscopic ear surgery, it is usually best to begin with surgeries that are likely to go well and lend themselves to the endoscopic approach. Once you have built up your skills, you will be better equipped to undertake more challenging surgeries using the endoscopic technique.

Patient Factors

It is often best to start with a simple operation such as the insertion of ventilation tubes or a simple underlay tympanoplasty. It would be unwise to start off with an endoscopic case that involves an extensive cholesteatoma. Likewise, choose a case that has a dry ear canal that is not full of granulation tissue and is uninfected, as this will make the surgery for easier and allow the basic principles of endoscopic ear surgery to be learned more quickly.

Disease Factors

Once you are familiar with the basics of raising a tympanomeatal flap and with accessing the middle ear, as well as with how instruments are used in the middle ear in endoscopic surgery, it is time to progress to cholesteatoma surgery. When selecting a case, it is well worth conducting preoperative computed tomography (CT) to assess the extent of the disease.

Disease limited to the mesotympanum or to the epitympanum lateral to the ossicular chain is the easiest to deal with, and this is also the case that an endoscopic surgeon should attempt when starting off. Cholesteatoma that extends into the mastoid is probably best undertaken using a combined approach with a mastoidectomy under a microscopic approach to the mastoid as well as an endoscopic approach to the middle ear. This approach is probably best kept in reserve until more experience has been obtained.

Although the endoscopic approaches afford a far better view of important structures, it does take time to get used to the way these are likely to appear in the operative field. This appearance will be very different from that of the microscopic approach, and for this reason it is important to ensure that the cases you begin with do not have any substantial anatomic variations or exposed structures, such as a fistula of the lateral semicircular canal or an obviously dehiscent facial nerve.

Surgical Factors

Figs. 2 through **10** show a series of steps, taken from several ear surgeries, demonstrating the basic technique of endoscopic ear surgery and the way the ear should look at each of these stages. **Fig. 3** shows the tympanomeatal flap being raised following canal incisions. Note the cottonoid pledgets that are being used to reduce bleeding from the cut edges of the flap. An important factor at this stage is the "fish-eye" nature of all endoscopes; the peripheries of the field are more magnified than the center. As a result of this optical effect, it is possible to misjudge the length of the tympanomeatal flap. The error is that the flap is usually made too short, and can become rolled up and difficult to replace on the ear canal. This misjudgment will also affect the integrity of the tympanic membrane and tympanomeatal flap if any bone is removed from the posterior canal wall or the scutum. Given this inherent bias, it is best to make the incision that joins the 2 radial incisions more lateral than one would expect. Having a slightly longer flap is not much of a hindrance in endoscopic ear surgery, as the access to the mesotympanum is so much larger that a carefully packed-off tympanomeatal flap will cause little interference with the surgical field. Much of the rest of the procedure takes place in the center of the endoscopic field

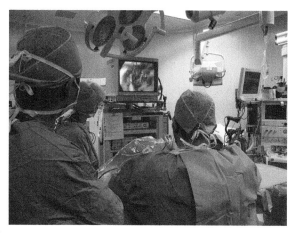

Fig. 2. Operating room setup.

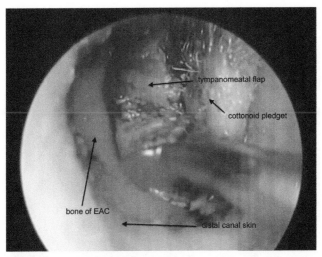

Fig. 3. Raising flap. EAC, external auditory canal.

and is not subject to this effect to any appreciable extent. **Fig. 4** shows the tympano-meatal flap raised to the level of the fibrous annulus, the middle ear having been entered; note how little bleeding takes place when careful injection of the field combined with careful dissection with cottonoid pledgets has been undertaken. Around the time that the middle ear has been entered, the lateral cut edge of the tympanomeatal flap stops bleeding and the medial edge is tucked away under a pledget, thus allowing good access to the middle ear in a bloodless field.

From here, further dissection and curettage of the overlying bone will expose the extent of the cholesteatoma and allow for it to be dissected under vision (see **Fig. 5**). Here it will become apparent that only a small amount of bone must be removed to provide a very wide view of the posterior mesotympanum and epitympanum.

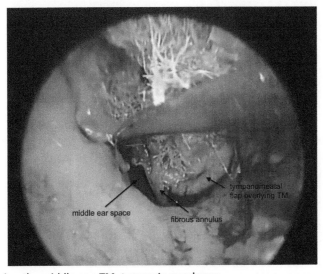

Fig. 4. Entering the middle ear. TM, tympanic membrane.

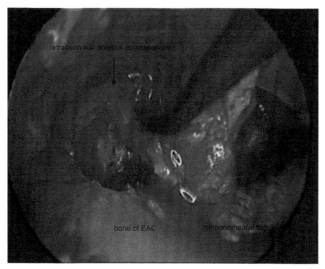

Fig. 5. Removing pocket. EAC, external auditory canal; TM, tympanic membrane.

Larger instruments such as malleus head shears can easily be passed alongside the endoscope to remove disease (see **Fig. 6**), and very accurate dissection can be performed as shown in **Fig. 7**, where cupped forceps are being used to remove disease from the capitellum of the stapes, and in **Fig. 8**, where cholesteatoma is being removed from the oval window where the footplate has been eroded.

Ossiculoplasty can be performed with little difficulty, using either autogenous tissue (see **Fig. 9**) or prostheses. These materials can be difficult to insert and manipulate when beginning, but the improved view soon outweighs the limitations of the technique.

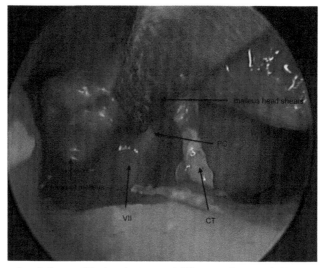

Fig. 6. Malleus head shears. CT, chorda tympani; PC, posterior canal; RWN, round window niche; VII, cranial nerve VII.

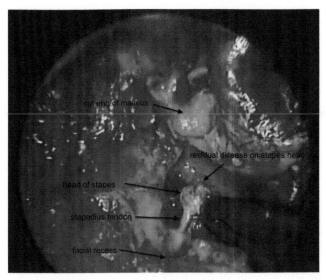

Fig. 7. Skin matrix from stapes.

Given that the skin lateral to the tympanomeatal flap incision has not been elevated, it remains in good condition relative to the same area where the ear has been retracted anteriorly (as with a postauricular incision) or posteriorly, as occurs in most endaural incisions. This factor, combined with the integrity of the tympanomeatal flap, allows for very accurate replacement of the skin of the ear canal after a graft has been inserted (see **Fig. 10**).

The smaller amount of bone that has been removed, combined with the improved integrity of the tympanomeatal flap in many cases, allows for almost all cases to only need a quantity of graft material that can be harvested from the tragus. A linear incision is made on the posterior surface of the tragus and the graft is harvested, leaving a thin buttress of cartilage on the lateral edge of the tragus to prevent cosmetic and functional deformities. Perichondrium alone, cartilage alone, or a composite of both can be used. A simple dressing for the ear such as an expansile wick is usually sufficient, and a head bandage is seldom required.

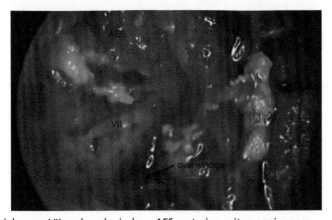

Fig. 8. Cranial nerve VII and oval window. AES, anterior epitympanic space.

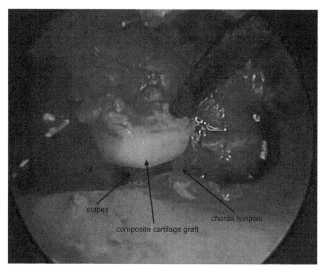

Fig. 9. Cartilage ossiculoplasty. VII, cranial nerve VII.

Investigations Before the Procedure

A high-resolution CT scan is useful before any middle ear procedure whereby the endoscopic approach is to be used. Standard axial, sagittal, and coronal views are not as helpful in the endoscopic setting as they are in the microscopic setting. The best series of views to use are those reconstructed along the plane of the external auditory meatus. These views allow the surgeon to visualize what will be encountered as the endoscope progresses.

Issues of Consent

Although the experienced endoscopic ear surgeon seldom needs to resort to a postauricular or endaural approach, it is vital to discuss whether more invasive surgery may need

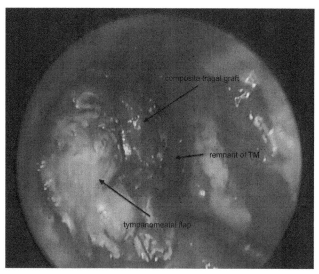

Fig. 10. Flaps replaced. TM, tympanic membrane.

to be undertaken should be endoscopic approach not be successful at first instance. Although patients are generally pleased to hear that there will be no scarring behind the ear, is quite routine to harvest perichondrium or cartilage graft from the tragus, mention of a small scar must be made to the patient before surgery is undertaken.

Preparing the Operating Room

The operating room can be set up in a fashion similar to that for standard ear surgery, with the exception that the microscope is replaced by an endoscope stack, which is usually positioned opposite the surgeon at eye level (see **Fig. 2**).

Preparing the Patient

The patient is prepared and draped in the usual fashion, with the ipsilateral shoulder being pulled down to allow easier access to the area. Instillation of local anesthetic/vasoconstrictor solution is particularly important in endoscopic ear surgery, as properly injecting the ear canal skin with a vasoconstrictive agent will reduce bleeding considerably.

Pitfalls

Giving up too soon
Hemorrhage
Narrow ear canal
Fogged endoscope

Giving up too early

Part of the philosophy of endoscopic surgery is the reduction of soft-tissue trauma required to access and remove abnormalities. Very little soft-tissue work is undertaken to reach the lesion in question and, as a result, the first surgical incision is the beginning of the tympanomeatal flap. Unlike traditional ear surgery, where this incision is sometimes made and then left while the postauricular incision is started, the canal incisions are made with the flap being lifted soon thereafter. This approach can sometimes cause bleeding, which makes raising the flap very difficult. It is at this stage that those new to the technique will consider that the advantages of endoscopic ear surgery are exaggerated and the difficulties far greater than expected. Unfortunately, at this initial stage the benefit of the endoscopic approach is not as evident as when the middle ear is reached (see **Fig. 4**). Once the initial challenge of the surgery has been overcome, the benefits of the wide field of view and improved access become obvious. It is important to get through the early part of the surgery to truly appreciate what endoscopic surgery of the ear has to offer.

Controlling hemorrhage

Other than the meticulous injection of vasoconstrictors mixed with local anesthetic into the ear canal skin, there are several very simple techniques that can be used to reduce the amount of bleeding when the tympanomeatal flap is raised (see **Fig. 3**). These techniques can be used throughout the operation, and should be used liberally to keep the operative field as free of blood as possible.

1. Cottonoid pledgets (neuro patties)

Using these pledgets soaked in epinephrine allows the surgeon to pack off areas of bleeding, and also to raise a tympanomeatal flap and maintain control of excess blood at the same time. As endoscopic surgery is currently largely a one-handed technique, it is often helpful to pack off the areas that are not being worked on so as to reduce the background ooze that may come from these surgical sites.

2. Saline flush/irrigation

Owing to the fact that endoscopic surgery is particularly vulnerable to "red-out," regular irrigation of the operative field washes away hemorrhage and provides the surgeon with a clean visual field that allows the surgeon to take advantage of the superior view afforded by the endoscope. Normal saline at body temperature stored in a 20-mL syringe with a soft catheter tip is the simplest way of providing irrigation.

3. Time

Once the surgeon is sufficiently familiar with endoscopic surgery, the amount of time saved during surgery is considerable, given that there is no soft-tissue approach and no need close the ear following surgery. In addition, far less healthy tissue is removed to reach disease in comparison with traditional approaches. The time saved needs to be invested. It is very easy to become overwhelmed during endoscopic surgery, as only a small amount of bleeding can become difficult to control and will affect the visual field far more than in standard ear surgery. The unfortunate aspect of the situation, however, is that the amount of bleeding is actually small but is considerably magnified by the endoscope. When increased hemorrhage arises, it is often best to pack the ear canal for 5 minutes and halt the surgery. This pause may be a good opportunity to harvest the graft material that may be required. On returning to the area once the packs are removed, the bleeding is usually completely settled. Taking time in endoscopic ear surgery is always rewarded.

Narrow canal

Undertaking endoscopic ear surgery through a narrow external auditory meatus can be very challenging, but there are several techniques that help considerably. In these cases it is useful to use a Lempert/endaural speculum to slightly dilate the ear canal and to massage excess infiltration from the canal skin. Once the tympanomeatal flaps have been raised, a curette can be used to enlarge the ear canal for improved access. Only a very small amount of bone needs to be removed to improve the access considerably when an endoscope is used.

Fogging of the endoscope

It is quite common for the endoscope to become fogged or misted with condensation, particularly at the beginning of the operation. Misting usually occurs because the endoscope is cold and the moist air found in the ear canal causes the tip of the lens to fog up. This problem can be solved by keeping the endoscope submerged in warm water before commencement of surgery. The use of a quality demisting solution (AntiFog) can be helpful once the surgery is under way.

GAINING SKILLS IN ENDOSCOPIC EAR SURGERY

The learning curve for endoscopic ear surgery is not as steep as that for microscopic surgery, as the microscope has been the mainstay of ear surgery for decades. Many experienced with endoscopy will find the technique easy to master, but surgeons who have limited themselves to an entirely microscopic otology practice are likely to find endoscopic ear surgery more difficult to perform. Despite this, with sufficient training and practice the technique is available to all. It is important to remember that the initial steps of the surgery are the most difficult, and these may be better started microscopically until the middle ear is reached, at which point the endoscope and its advantages can be used. Once comfortable with partial use of the endoscope, most surgeons will then progress to use the endoscope exclusively for indicated surgery.

The International Working Group on Endoscopic Ear Surgery runs several courses around the world to provide surgeons with the skills and techniques necessary to begin using the endoscope for transcanal endoscopic ear surgery. Although not essential, these courses allow the surgeon to gain the necessary technical skills required to begin endoscopic ear surgery immediately, and are recommended to anyone wishing to use this technique.

International Working Group on Endoscopic Ear Surgery: www.iwgees.org.

Index

Note: Page numbers of article titles are in **boldface** type.

Otolaryngol Clin N Am 46 (2013) 257–260
http://dx.doi.org/10.1016/S0030-6665(13)00012-1
0030-6665/13/$ – see front matter © 2013 Elsevier Inc. All rights reserved.

oto.theclinics.com

Moving?

Make sure your subscription moves with you!

To notify us of your new address, find your **Clinics Account Number** (located on your mailing label above your name), and contact customer service at:

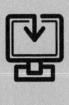

Email: journalscustomerservice-usa@elsevier.com

800-654-2452 (subscribers in the U.S. & Canada)
314-447-8871 (subscribers outside of the U.S. & Canada)

Fax number: 314-447-8029

Elsevier Health Sciences Division
Subscription Customer Service
3251 Riverport Lane
Maryland Heights, MO 63043

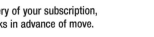

*To ensure uninterrupted delivery of your subscription, please notify us at least 4 weeks in advance of move.

Printed and bound by CPI Group (UK) Ltd, Croydon, CR0 4YY

03/10/2024

01040439-0017